# Table of Contents

## Section A – THE BASICS

## SECTION B - SITUATIONS

## SECTION C - ATTITUDES & EMOTIONS

## Introduction

Being a teen can be a lot of fun, a little bit confusing and awkward, and sometimes completely challenging. It's not always easy being a teen. And having food allergies does not make it any easier.

As a teen, you are expected to take on more responsibilities, face new situations, and make important decisions. As a teen with food allergies, there is the additional challenge of taking control of your own health condition under a new set of circumstances. Luckily, there are a lot of other teens going through the same things you are!

Remember when you were a kid and things seemed so simple? Your parents and other adults around you probably did much of the work keeping you safe with your allergies while you learned some of the basic skills like carrying your epinephrine auto-injector (like EpiPen®, Allerject®/Auvi-Q®), reading food labels, and telling people what you were allergic to. Now, it's definitely not that easy. But having allergies can also be very manageable—provided you know how to approach new situations.

Throughout your teenage years, you will face challenges such as changing schools, getting a job, dating for the first time, travelling without your parents, and planning ahead for your future. As teenagers, we often go to friends for advice when dealing with these new types of challenges. But how many of your friends have felt unsafe at a potluck because of food being shared, had trouble emotionally recovering after an allergic reaction or experienced being teased or bullied simply because of a food allergy? If you've had allergic reactions, or felt sheer frustration because your allergies have made you feel excluded, anxious or scared, you are not alone.

Having allergies is a part of who you are. Yet it does not have to define you. It does not have to prevent you from experiencing your teenage years just like everyone else.

We have compiled stories from teens and young adults with food allergies who offer advice and tips on handling different situations and emotions. Although you may have never met our youth contributors, it's our hope that you can relate to their stories and gain insight and support from their experiences. Not every chapter may apply to you right now, but the information will hopefully help prepare you for handling future situations.

Although the main focus of this book is food allergies, teens with allergies to non-food related items (like medication, latex or insect stings), intolerances, sensitivities or other health conditions can appreciate the stories and tips shared throughout. Many of the key lessons are universal and we encourage you to share with your friends, family, and others who may benefit from them. Also, remember that we all have different perceptions of risk and ways to handle food allergies that work best for us. Although there are some non-negotiable things like always carrying your medication, there is no perfect script for asking a waiter about ingredients or telling a new friend about an allergy. We hope the stories within will help provide perspective as you develop your own tactics, comfort level, and style.

We titled this book a "Guidebook" because we hope it will help guide you through the challenges and situations you will face when managing allergies on your own while living a normal teenage life.

Your allergic friends and book editors,
Kyle and Daniela


## Contributors


This book was made possible through a grant from TD Securities and proceeds from the Annual Sean Delaney Memorial Golf Classic. Their generous support to Food Allergy Canada (formerly

Anaphylaxis Canada) has allowed us to focus our efforts on making life easier for teens and young adults with food allergies.

With every single resource or project we create for teens, we consult and work with a team of allergic youth from across Canada. This book features their stories and advice from their experiences. Male or female, 13 or 21, we think that the stories and tips in this book will be relatable and helpful for all youth with food allergies.

**Illustrations:**

Katelyn Gerke
Mick MacEachern

**Book Contributors:**

Arianne Kirkey (25) – Allergies: Peanuts, tree nuts, eggs, fish and sesame

Bailey Francis (18) - Allergies: Peanuts, tree nuts and chickpeas

Caitlin Finnerty (23) - Allergies: Peanuts, tree nuts, milk, eggs and shellfish

Caitlyn Pirker (22) - Allergies: Peanuts, tree nuts, eggs and wheat

Chelsea Vineyard (20) - Allergies: Peanuts and penicillin

Dylan Brennan (24) - Allergies: Peanuts and tree nuts

Emily Rose Belbin (16) - Allergies: Peanuts and tree nuts

Erika Ladouceur (25) - Allergies: Peanuts, tree nuts, soy, legumes, wheat, penicillin and sulpha

Giulia Cavaleri (21) - Allergies: Peanuts, tree nuts, fish and shellfish

Hannah Lank (17) - Allergies: Peanuts and tree nuts

Harrison Ho-Tom (18) - Allergies: Dairy, eggs, tree nuts, fish, shellfish, soy, sesame, apples, pears and cherries

Jazmin Chase (21) - Allergies: Peanuts, tree nuts, milk, eggs, soy and latex

Karen De Leon (20) - Allergies: Peanuts, tree nuts and soy

Katelyn Gerke (23) - Allergies: Peanuts, tree nuts, peas, chickpeas and lentils

Lindsay Schnarr (22) - Allergies: Peanuts, tree nuts, soy and lactose intolerant

Mathew Keating (22) - Allergies: Peanuts, tree nuts, and milk

Michelle Davidson (19) - Allergies: Peanuts

Nick Pothier (21) - Allergies: Peanuts and tree nuts

Nicole Kovac (23) - Allergies: Peanuts, tree nuts, fish, shellfish, crustaceans, sesame, peas and beans

Samantha Steiner-Mayman (15) - Allergies: Peanuts, mustard and kiwi

Sebastian Blokowski (16) - Allergies: Peanuts, tree nuts and penicillin

Shayna Rak (18) - Allergies: Peanuts, tree nuts, sesame, wheat, pumpkin seeds and kiwi

Sophia Biro (22) - Allergies: Pumpkin seeds

Stephanie Kwolek (24) - Allergies: Peanuts, tree nuts; exercise-induced with unknown triggers

Sydney Harris (18) - Allergies: Pineapple, coconut, strawberries and cashews

Sydney Proudfoot (21) - Allergies: Peanuts, tree nuts, mushroom and lactose intolerant

Talia Aboud (23) - Allergies: Milk, tree nuts, fish, sesame, mustard, kiwi and legumes

Tess Bantock (25) - Allergies: Peanuts and tree nuts

**Book Editors:**

Kyle Dine - Working with Food Allergy Canada (formerly Anaphylaxis Canada) since 2008, Kyle has been involved in many allergy education and awareness projects for youth. He has created educational music about food allergies and tours across North America presenting school assemblies and performing at special events. He has multiple food allergies and stays positive with his motto "Food Allergies Rock!"

Daniela Deschamps - Daniela is a 3rd year Mechanical Engineering student at Queen's University (Ontario) with several allergies including peanut, tree nuts, legumes and seeds. Her interests include playing sports, especially rowing and rugby, travelling, hanging out with friends, and leading white-water canoe trips at summer camp. By planning ahead and taking precautions, Daniela has never let allergies stop her from doing what she loves!

Aaron Sutherland - Aaron is a freelance writer and editor who also happens to have allergies. Growing up with potentially life-threatening allergies is not always easy. It is his hope that this e-book will make life a little easier for current and future teens with allergies. He became involved with this project because he knows first-hand how much stress and time a resource like this would have saved him were it around when he was a teenager.

**Medical Review provided by Dr. Anne Ellis**

Dr. Anne Ellis, Associate Professor and Chair, Division of Allergy & Immunology, Department of Medicine, Queen's University, Kingston, ON. Twitter: @DrAnneEllis.

**Review Team**
Laura Bantock, Director, Western Region, Food Allergy Canada
Laurie Harada, Executive Director, Food Allergy Canada
Marilyn Allen
Anne Borden
Tracy Bush

Susan Hawrylow

Aileen Li

Andrew Au

Daniel Loberto

Karen DeLeon

Stephanie Kwolek

Samantha Steiner-Maynem

**Additional Resources**

Food Allergy Canada – www.foodallergycanada.ca
On Facebook www.facebook.com/foodallergycanada
On Twitter – www.twitter.com/foodallergycan
On YouTube – www.youtube.com/foodallergycanada
Why Risk It? Allergy Resources for Youth – www.whyriskit.ca
Health Canada - http://www.hc-sc.gc.ca/fn-an/securit/allerg/fa-aa/index-eng.php
EpiPen® - www.epipen.ca
Allerject® - www.allerject.ca

**Disclaimer**

The information provided in this book is for reference and educational purposes and is not a substitute for medical advice or care. This book was designed to support, not replace, the relationship that exists between readers and their existing physicians.

The material in this book was written to provide a guideline for care and wellbeing. Food Allergy Canada disclaims any responsibility for any adverse effects resulting from the information presented in this book. The information enclosed is not designed to take the place of a doctor's instructions. Individuals are urged to contact a doctor for specific information regarding guidelines for care. The inclusion of brand name medications or medical devices does not imply endorsement by Food Allergy Canada. The personal stories and views expressed within do not necessarily reflect those of Food Allergy Canada.

**Copyright**
Food Allergy Canada © 2015
ISBN: 9781483557137

## Dedication

This book is dedicated to all youth with food allergies. The path to a cure is currently uncertain, but the knowledge to thrive with allergies is known.

# Section A

# The Basics

# Chapter 1
*What are Allergies?*

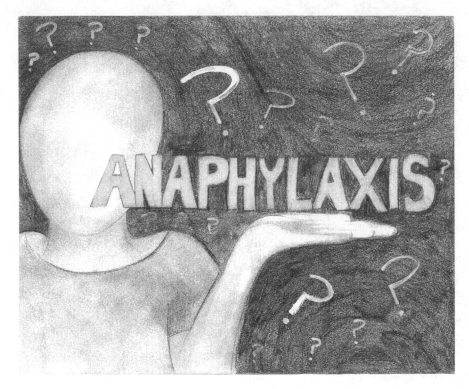

## Introduction

If you have food allergies, this topic hardly needs an introduction. You know all too well what they are, what they can do to you, and the importance of avoiding the things that you are allergic to. Did you know, however, that food allergies affect approximately 2.5 million Canadians?[1] You are definitely not alone.

Anaphylaxis is not only a hard word to say or spell. It's also a hard concept to understand. Many people who are not very aware of food allergies think that they only cause sniffles or sneezing. Anaphylaxis is a serious allergic reaction that can happen quickly and is potentially life-threatening.

---

[1] L. Soller et al. *Overall Prevalence of Self-reported Food Allergy in Canada*, Journal of Allergy and Clinical Immunology (2012). doi: 10.1016/j.jaci.2012.06.029

There is no cure for food allergies and even trace amounts of an allergen can cause a severe reaction. This is why it's so important for people with serious food allergies to know how to avoid the things they are allergic to and to have epinephrine (like EpiPen® or Allerject®/Auvi-Q™) with them at all times.

*Quick Tip – According to recent studies in the US, it appears that the incidence of peanut and tree nut allergies among children has tripled from 1997 to 2008.*[2]

## What would you say? (Q&A)

*Q&A with YAP members Hannah, Sydney H., Talia, and Tess*

**How long have you had allergies?**

**Hannah** – I've had allergies since I was diagnosed at age 2.

**Sydney H.** - I was diagnosed with food allergies when I was 14.

**Talia** - I've had allergies my whole life!

**Tess** - I had my first allergic reaction when I was 15 months old. I was officially diagnosed about three months later. I had something called panel testing done and my parents were told that I had multiple food allergies. For approximately 13 years, I avoided many food groups because I believed that I was allergic to them. Thanks to a new allergist, and multiple oral challenges, he disproved many of these and narrowed this list down to peanuts and tree nuts. I have a much wider diet now!

---

[2] Branum AM & Lukacs SL. *Food Allergy Among U.S. Children: Trends in Prevalence and Hospitalizations,* National Center for Health Statistics, Hyattsville, MD, 2008

## How many people do you know at school with allergies?

**Hannah** - Throughout my life, I've known very few other people who have allergies as serious as my own. At my high school, I know of only 5 other people who have a food allergy.

**Sydney H.** - I know about half a dozen people at my school with food allergies. But I'm always looking to meet more!

**Talia -** A few of my friends have seasonal allergies. But only two of them have food allergies.

**Tess** - I know at least ten people who have food allergies at my university. Since moving to Vancouver, I have made two very good girl friends. Both of them have a variety of food allergies as well! I guess birds of a feather really do flock together!


## What's the toughest part about having allergies?

**Hannah** - For me, the toughest part about having allergies is the extra effort I must exert to ensure the food I eat is safe. Other people don't have to worry about travelling to another country and communicating their dietary needs or asking their friend's mom if the birthday cake she baked is allergen-free. I never put something in my mouth without first reading its ingredients, asking someone if it's safe, and/or examining it in great detail.

**Sydney H.** - The toughest part about my allergies is feeling excluded at social events.

**Talia** - Going to dinners with friends can be tricky. I'm lucky to have really understanding friends who often let me choose the restaurant so I feel more comfortable.

**Tess -** I think the toughest thing about having food allergies is explaining it to other people and having them really 'get it'. I think that's what I have struggled with the most over the years. For some people, it just clicks and they seem to really grasp the seriousness of it. And, for others, it just doesn't.

**How do you typically explain what allergies are to others?**

**Hannah -** If someone does not know what allergies are, I generally describe them as a health condition that results in a person not being able to eat certain foods because it could lead to a severe reaction throughout the body.

**Sydney H.** - I find that the majority of people nowadays understand what allergies are. However, if they don't, I typically tell them that my body simply recognizes the allergen as a germ, bacteria or disease that it tries to fight against. I explain that this can have disastrous consequences.

**Talia** – Sometimes, to explain cross-contamination, I compare an allergen to something dangerous. I ask, would your friends feel comfortable eating a candy bar that said "may contain rat poison" on the label? Probably not, given that it could be dangerous to their health like an allergen can be for me.

**Tess** - I try to keep it simple and to the point without excluding the seriousness of my food allergies. I usually say something like "I have a food allergy and I'm allergic to x, y, z. This means that, if I ingest x, y, z, my life could be at risk." Sometimes, if people ask, I'll tell them what kind of symptoms I could experience. I typically concentrate on airway and blood pressure symptoms, how it feels, and maybe explain a past experience or two. I find that most people who ask questions are genuinely interested in what happens during a reaction and what has to take place in terms of treatment. It's always nice to show people an auto-injector. It spreads knowledge about allergies and it's sometimes a good opportunity to dispel some of the myths about allergies that are out there.

## Summary Tips

1) Anaphylaxis is a serious, potentially life-threatening allergic reaction.

2) Statistics show that more and more people are getting food allergies.

3) Approximately 7% of Canadians self-report a food allergy.[3]

---

[3] L. Soller et al. *Overall Prevalence of Self-reported Food Allergy in Canada*, Journal of Allergy and Clinical Immunology (2012). doi: 10.1016/j.jaci.2012.06.029

# Chapter 2
## *Common Causes*

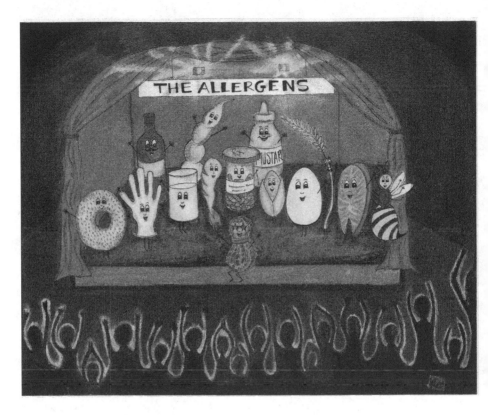

## Introduction

Peanuts, peanuts, PEANUTS! With all of the attention peanut allergy gets, you'd think all other allergens were either non-existent or just not as serious. Although peanut allergy can be serious, so can ALL food allergies!

People can be allergic to many foods and substances. However, in Canada, 10 allergens are determined as "priority allergens" by Health Canada because of their prevalence and reaction severity, among other factors. These priority allergens are:

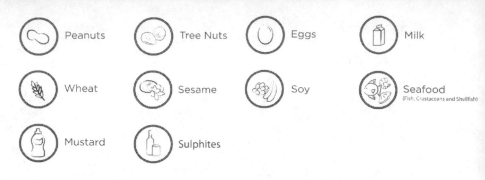

## Note about Sulphites

*Sulphites are food additives used as preservatives to maintain food colour and prolong shelf-life. Although sulphites do not cause a true allergic reaction, sulphite-sensitive people may experience similar reactions as those with food allergies, or may have other adverse symptoms.*

These priority allergens have special rules when it comes to ingredient labelling. You can learn about them in the "Reading Ingredients" chapter.

But allergies don't just stop at foods. Other common causes include medicine (such as penicillin and amoxicillin), latex (commonly found in medical gloves, balloons, and condoms), and insect venom (bee stings and ant bites).

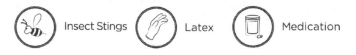

Although rare, exercise-induced anaphylaxis is a real issue where the exertion from exercise can trigger symptoms when combined with a specific food. There is another cause, which is quite complex, called "idiopathic anaphylaxis", where there is no known trigger.

*Quick Tip* - *Remember, allergists have the tests and knowledge needed to properly diagnose allergies.*

## What would you say? (Q&A)
*Arianne, Hannah, and Nicole*

### What's one allergy you wish you could trade?

**Arianne** - One allergy I wish I could trade would be my freshwater fish allergy. It is the most recent allergy that I've developed. It has been hard to come to terms with it since I had previously enjoyed fish as a healthy meal. But I've since learned to look for other options with similar nutrients.

**Hannah** - I wish that I was allergic to shellfish and not tree nuts. Shellfish aren't often listed as a 'may contain' food and I don't like shrimp anyway!

**Nicole** - Tough call! I love desserts and sweets. So I would definitely change the peanut and nut allergies. Then I could eat all the chocolate and desserts I want!

### Do you ever find your allergens hidden in certain foods or products? What are they?

**Arianne –** I was recently on the hunt for a new kind of juice to add to a summer punch. One day I saw delicious looking blood-orange lemonade at the store. As I skimmed the ingredients, I was shocked to see that, at the end of the list, there was a statement saying "Contains: Tree Nuts." I immediately put it down and realized I have to be more careful when reading ingredients—even in the most harmless foods or drinks.

**Hannah** - Usually peanuts and tree nuts are clearly listed as an ingredient in a particular food. But once I was about to buy a pie to bake at home and realized that one of the ingredients was almond extract! I had even bought that brand of pie before. However, they must have changed the ingredients. It was a good thing that I decided to re-read the ingredient list. It just proves that your allergens can pop-up in the ingredients of certain foods when you're least expecting it.

**Nicole** - I always find it odd when I find fish (anchovy paste) in certain sauces and dressings. I have learned to double-check these items!

**Do you think it is much harder to have multiple allergies versus only one?**

**Arianne** - I think it is harder to have more than one allergy. Being vigilant about multiple food allergies is challenging. I've often felt self-conscious and like a burden when I list all my allergens to friends or servers at restaurants. I just have to be confident that all of my allergies are important and need to be known in all situations.

**Hannah** - Although I don't have a lot of food allergies, I think it would be difficult to be allergic to peanuts, tree nuts, AND milk, for example, because then you can't drink almond milk and you're even MORE limited when it comes to your food choices. That being said, it certainly isn't impossible to manage—everyone adjusts to what they're given.

**Nicole** – Ummmm...that depends on the allergy I guess. And where you live. If you were only allergic to seafood, but you happened to live in a coastal area, that would be more challenging than being allergic to multiple foods that are not from your region.

**A lot of focus is placed on what you *can't* eat. But what are your favourite things you *can* eat?**

**Arianne** - Dairy products, wheat products, and fruit. With the large amount of allergies I have, I am glad that I don't have to find substitutes for everything. But thankfully many exist.

**Hannah** – I love bread and tropical fruits like papayas, mangos, and pineapple!

**Nicole** – Chocolate, CHOCOLATE, and Cheese!

## Summary Tips

1) There are 10 "priority food allergens" in Canada that are known to be the most common.

2) Insect stings, latex, and medications can also cause allergic reactions.

3) Although some allergens are more common than others, any food can potentially be an allergen.

# Chapter 3

*Symptoms*

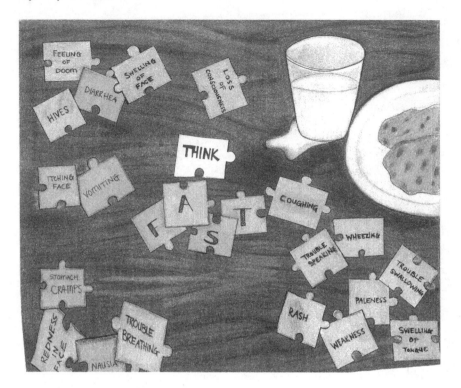

## Introduction

Naming all of the symptoms of an allergic reaction on paper can help people, especially the non-allergic, remember them.

If you have allergies, however, you know the feeling you get when something isn't right. Whether it's a visible symptom on your skin, or pain and/or constriction on the inside, you know something bad is happening. And your mind becomes focused on it.

A serious allergic reaction can start within minutes of coming into contact with an allergy trigger—or hours after the fact. They may include any or all of these symptoms. Know how to spot the signs and remember them by this handy acronym: **Think "FAST."**

## THINK "FAST"

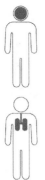

**Face**
itching,
redness,
swelling

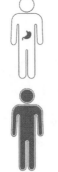

**Stomach**
pain,
vomiting,
diarrhea,
nausea

**Airway**
trouble breathing,
coughing, wheezing,
trouble swallowing
and speaking

**Total body**
hives, rash,
weakness, paleness,
sense of doom, loss
of consciousness

**Other:** dizziness, pale/blue colour

It's important to note that these symptoms happen independently of each other and may be different from one reaction to the next.

Knowing how these symptoms feel is important. We've asked members of our youth panel to describe what they felt in these situations.

*"It really felt like my world was collapsing in the pit of my stomach."*

*"Metallic taste in my mouth."*

*"I knew something was very wrong and it took me a few seconds to piece together the symptoms and conclude that I was actually having an allergic reaction."*

*"It started with a tingling sensation on my tongue and lips that quickly moved to tightness throughout my mouth and throat. It all happened so quickly."*

Most importantly, when you feel any of these symptoms, and suspect it might be an allergic reaction, seek help immediately and do not isolate yourself. Be prepared to treat your reaction. You will learn more about this in the next chapter.

*Quick Tip - A biphasic reaction is when the symptoms of an allergic reaction reappear after the initial treatment. This is why it's so important to get to the hospital to make sure the reaction is completely gone.*

## What would you say? (Q&A)
*Emily Rose, Giulia, and Lindsay*

**Do your reactions always have the same symptoms or are they different?**

**Emily Rose** - Most of the time my reactions start with the same symptoms. Usually I notice that I am having a reaction when my mouth feels tight. After that I usually get itchy in my throat and around my ears.

**Giulia –** No, my reactions almost never have the same symptoms. It really depends on the allergen I accidentally ingested and the severity of my allergy to that particular food. For example, I'm not as allergic to almonds as I would be to hazelnuts. When I accidentally ingested a food containing almonds, when I was younger, I broke out in hives and my skin started to turn red. Only after those symptoms emerged did I start feeling other systems including shortness of breath and breathing difficulties. When I accidentally ingested a hazelnut one time, I did not get any of the usual "symptoms" of an allergic reaction. I started vomiting immediately and found that I had trouble swallowing.

**Lindsay** - My reactions typically have the same symptoms: an itchy throat and hives around my mouth.

**What symptom do you find the scariest?**

**Emily Rose** - This has only happened to me a few times. The scariest symptom is when my blood pressure drops. It is one of the strangest feelings. My vision starts to go dark and I feel light-headed. I end up unable to hear aside from a ringing in my ears.

**Giulia** - I find shortness of breath the most frightening symptom. It feels as if you are drowning. You desperately want to take a deep breath. But your body is preventing you from doing that.

**Lindsay** - I find having an itchy throat the scariest because I know this is a sign that my airway could close very quickly.

**At what age did you start to fully understand how serious your allergies were? How did that make you feel?**

**Emily Rose** - I realized the severity of my allergy when I was about eight. This was when Sabrina's Law came out in Ontario. At first, I found it strange that I had to carry my auto-injector everywhere with me. My mom used the truth to explain why. If I ate peanuts, I could have a life-threatening reaction. When I was eight, my parents also started to teach me how to handle my allergy independently. At first, I was very scared. I think that helped me in some ways. I was kept 'on my toes' and never took risks.

**Giulia** - I think I realized the severity of my allergies from a really young age. My mom always made sure to emphasize the importance of keeping my auto-injector with me at all times and the importance of never ever eating anyone else's food. I wouldn't say she instilled fear in me in terms of making sure I was aware of the severity of my allergies. But it definitely made me more mature than the other kids around me. I was always reading labels and checking before I put anything in my mouth whereas other children could eat whatever they wanted.

**Lindsay** – I realized the severity of my allergies around the age of 6 when I was entering elementary school. This was also when I became responsible for carrying my own auto-injector. This made me feel different and isolated at times.

**Have you ever had a "biphasic reaction" where the symptoms came back after initial treatment?**

**Emily Rose** – No I haven't.

**Giulia** - Yes, I've had a biphasic reaction once in my life. After the initial allergic reaction, and the administration of epinephrine, I had thought that calling the ambulance was unnecessary because I was feeling better. Around 40 minutes later, my previous symptoms had returned and intensified.

**Lindsay** - Luckily I have not!

**When do you know that it's really an allergic reaction? Is it hard to tell?**

**Emily Rose** – I start to feel a tightening feeling in my mouth. This is usually shortly followed by other symptoms.

**Giulia** - My allergist told me a helpful tip that I keep in mind. He told me that, if you are having more than one symptom at the same time, it is likely an allergic reaction. If you puke, for example, it may not be a symptom of an allergic reaction. But, if you puke and are experiencing shortness of breath or red, itchy skin, it is most likely an allergic reaction, and I know I should take it seriously.

**Lindsay** - I know that it is really an allergic reaction when my initial symptoms don't go away after drinking some water and a few minutes has passed. It can be hard to tell. But, once you know, you know!

## Summary Tips

1) Remember to Think "**FAST**" to remember the symptoms that happen to the **F**ace, **A**irway, **S**tomach, and **T**otal body.
2) Symptoms can happen within minutes of coming into contact with your allergen.
3) A "biphasic reaction" is when the symptoms reappear after the initial treatment. They can occur up to several hours afterwards.

# Chapter 4
## *Treatment*

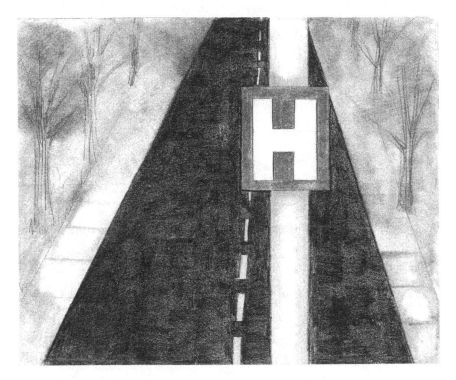

## Introduction

Many of us have received conflicting information about how to treat allergic reactions. This may be, in part, because of how guidelines have changed over time. Doctors continue to learn more about anaphylaxis as more data on the most effective treatments emerges. You may have also heard about potential "cures" for allergies. While there is a lot of research being done, and there are many interesting ideas out there, there is currently no cure. We will, however, talk a bit about what is being tried and what may work in the future.

**In terms of current treatment for anaphylaxis, epinephrine auto-injectors are the way to go. Epinephrine first. Period. There should be no "wait-and-see" approach, no treating with an anti-histamine first, and no chugging of water with the hope that the reaction will subside.**

Anaphylaxis happens so quickly. And epinephrine is the only proven way to stop it in its tracks.

Let's address the elephant in the room—needles. Does an auto-injector hurt? Well, yes. But surprisingly less than you would probably expect if you've never used one. It's a tiny prick. This pales in comparison to how the other symptoms are attacking your body. Often, the more difficult aspect of using an auto-injector is that it makes the entire issue seem more serious. You could be injecting yourself with a needle at the dinner table, for example.

Yes, 9-1-1, or your local emergency service, must be called. You will have to go to the hospital for monitoring. But isn't it worth it when compared to the alternative? Sure you might be the centre of attention that day and you may feel embarrassed by it. So what? You would be more embarrassed if you tried to ignore the reaction and kept it a secret from others until things were out of control. People will want to help you. They will be there to support you. They will be there for you that much more afterward to help make sure it never happens again.

In Canada, we currently have two auto-injectors available: EpiPen® and Allerject®.

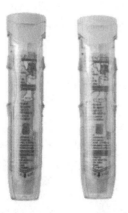 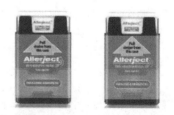

**EpiPen® (Pfizer Canada)**
**0.15 mg / 0.30 mg**

**Allerject® (Sanofi Canada)**
**0.15 mg / 0.30 mg**

Which one you carry is up to you. Just carry it, okay? Also remember to have two doses with you in case the symptoms are not gone or getting worse. An extra dose also gives you more time to get to a hospital for proper treatment.

It's very exciting to know that a lot of research is currently being done about treatments for food allergies. Research for treatments such as immunotherapy, among others, is in progress. As mentioned earlier, it's important to remember that there is currently no cure for food allergies. Below is a list of current research being done. Be sure to ask your allergist if you're interested in learning more.

**Oral Immunotherapy (OIT)**[4] – A tiny amount of the allergen (for example, peanut flour) is given under close medical supervision. The amount of allergen is increased over time with reactions that are monitored and treated. Studies suggest a definite increase in the amount of allergen a person can tolerate being exposed to with this treatment, but so far, everyone has reactions during the therapy. Research is currently being conducted to see if treatment can result in long-term tolerance rather than just short-term relief (desensitization).

**Sublingual Immunotherapy (SLIT)**[5] - This treatment involves placing a small amount of the allergen, dissolved in a solution, under the tongue for one or two minutes. It is done under close medical supervision. The results show that short-term relief can be achieved. But more studies must be done to assess long-term tolerance.

**Epicutaneous Immunotherapy (ET)**[6] – In a similar approach to the nicotine patch, a small patch is placed on the skin and releases a small quantity of the allergen over time in hopes of building

---

[4] Virkud YV, Vickery BP. *Advances in immunotherapy for food allergy*. Discov Med. 2012.

[5] Virkud YV, Vickery BP. *Advances in immunotherapy for food allergy*. Discov Med. 2012.

[6] Medical Daily. *Viaskin Peanut Patch Renews Hope for Allergic Kids: The Future of Skin-Based Treatments*. http://www.medicaldaily.com/viaskin-peanut-patch-renews-hope-allergic-kids-future-skin-based-treatments-323270. Accessed: 25 February, 2015.

tolerance. There have been promising results with "peanut patches" and more research is being done to include treatment for other allergens, including milk.

**Chinese Herbal Medicine**[7] - Ongoing studies are being conducted regarding the safety and effectiveness of a Chinese herbal formula, FAHF-2, to prevent serious, life-threatening allergic reactions. This herbal formula has been tested in a study involving patients with peanut and tree nut allergies. It was determined to be safe and well-tolerated. Current clinical trials include peanut, tree nut, fish, shellfish, and sesame allergies.

**Anti-IgE Therapy**[8] - A medicine for the treatment of asthma is being studied as a possible short-term relief treatment for food allergies. It consists of anti-IgE molecules that bind to IgE—the antibody involved in allergic reactions. Researchers hope to be able to determine whether this medication could prevent allergic reactions. Current research is focused on combining the treatment with OIT to possibly create long-term tolerance.

Hopefully scientists will soon be able to pinpoint what actually causes allergies, why they are increasing in prevalence, and how they can be cured. In the meantime, it's important to learn how to avoid and manage your allergies as well as how to use your auto-injector in the case of an emergency.

*Quick Tip* - *There **are** proven immunotherapy treatments available for some people allergic to things like insect stings, pollen, and pet dander. Immunotherapy for stinging insects in particular is highly effective, and can reduce your risk of anaphylaxis from about 50% down to 3%. Check with your allergist for more information.*

---

[7] [8] Virkud YV, Vickery BP. *Advances in immunotherapy for food allergy.* Discov Med. 2012.

## What would you say? (Q&A)

*Lindsay, Sophia, Sydney P.*

### Where do you carry your EpiPen® or Allerject®?

**Lindsay** - If I am at school, my EpiPen® will be in the front pocket of my backpack where it is easily accessible. When I am going out, it will be in a purse or in my pocket.

**Sydney P.** - It really depends on the season! In the winter, I carry my auto-injector in my jacket pocket. In the summer, I usually carry it in a purse. At all times, I always carry a second auto-injector in a small front pocket on my backpack. And all of my friends know which pocket it is!

### What do you do if you forget it?

**Lindsay** - If I forget my EpiPen®, the majority of the time I will avoid eating anything.

**Sophia** – Ideally, I would try not to eat anything until I can go home and get it. It's always better to be safe than sorry!

**Sydney P.** - The answer to this question would almost always be "turn around and go get it." However, if I am travelling a long way from home, I always carry an extra prescription just in case!

### How many times have you used your auto-injector?

**Lindsay** - Thankfully I have never had to use it!

**Sophia** - I have used my auto-injector twice in my life. Both times were in the last couple of years. Once I even used it at my own house!

**Sydney P.** - I have used my auto-injector 4 times in the past 8 years. But I am currently on a two and a half year reaction–free streak!

**At what point during the reaction have you given yourself epinephrine?**

Kyle - I'll admit that I haven't always given myself epinephrine when I should have. It's intimidating to use a needle. As you know, once you do, you've pressed the "panic button" and you'll need to go to the hospital. I now know how important it is to use it upon the first signs of anaphylaxis. It's just not worth waiting to see how far it progresses.

Sophia - I gave myself epinephrine about thirty seconds after I realized something was not right. I was panicking at first. But I came to my senses and knew it I had to do it immediately.

Sydney P. - I usually give myself my auto-injector upon the first signs of an allergic reaction—which, for me, is a tingling on my tongue.

**Would you ever be nervous or scared to use your epinephrine? Why?**

Lindsay - I think I might be a little nervous because it's a needle. But I know that this is a life or death situation and I must use my auto-injector to help save my life.

Sophia - I was incredibly nervous the first time I had to use my auto-injector. I was home alone and, even though I was nineteen, I had never imagined what it would be like. It's not only the feeling of having to inject yourself. It's the feeling of what's going to happen after. You know what you have to do even if you are nervous.

Sydney P. - I was very nervous to give myself my auto-injector the first time I had an allergic reaction. I didn't want to make the trip to the hospital if I wasn't having a true reaction. That said, I've learned that it's much better to use it than to wait until things have progressed to a dangerous level. It seems to me that the earlier I administer the auto-injector, the less time I have to spend in the hospital!

**Does it hurt?**

**Sophia** – As much as I hate needles, I really don't remember it hurting at all! When you're in a situation that requires you to use the auto-injector to begin with, the thought of the needle isn't as terrifying as some might make it out to be.

**Sydney P.** - To be completely honest, it really doesn't hurt. I think the flu shot hurts more! Don't be fooled by the giant shape of the whole device. The needle is actually very tiny. I was very afraid that it would hurt the first time I had a reaction. So I asked someone else to administer my auto-injector for me. But, after realizing how easy it was, I now do it myself!

Summary Tips

1) Epinephrine is the first line treatment for an anaphylactic reaction.
2) Never keep a reaction to yourself. Tell someone and get help right away.
3) There is currently no cure. But research continues to be done to find a treatment.

# Chapter 5
## *Reading Ingredients*

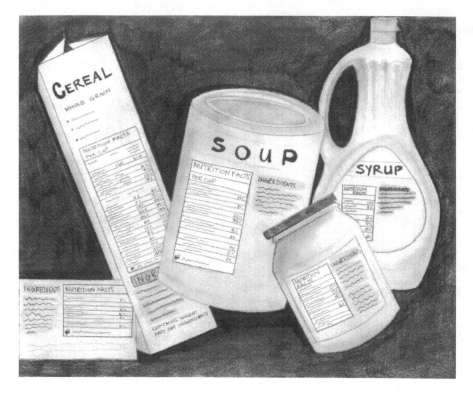

## Introduction

If you've had food allergies for most of your life, reading ingredients probably seems like second nature to you. You flip the package over, read the list, and pay extra attention to any wording that highlights the allergens inside. Then you double-check the package for anything you may have missed. You may be so good at it that you can pick out an allergen within just a couple of seconds. Sometimes it might seem like a hassle to have to read every label (such as when a friend bakes you something and you have to go digging through the garbage to find the wrapper). But, trust us, it's worth it. Then there are also the precautionary warnings saying "may contain" or "made in a facility that also processes..." (or some other variation of the phrase). **It is strongly recommended that you do not eat any foods with these warnings.**

For anyone new to reading labels, or as a reminder that may be useful when teaching friends and family how to read labels, there are a number of considerations aside from simply what is in the ingredients list. It is essential to be able to recognize different names for your allergen. For example, if you are allergic to milk, you should be aware that both "whey" and "casein" would not be safe. It is also important to know which forms of an allergen may be okay for you. For example, if you are allergic to soy protein, you may be able to tolerate soybean oil, soy lecithin or other forms of soy. But this is a decision you should discuss with your allergist.

When it comes to precautionary labels (e.g. "may contain" statements), it is important to realize that these terms are put on by a manufacturer to tell you that an allergen might have unintentionally got into a mixture or come in contact with another allergen during or before the production process. This is a voluntary step that manufacturers can use to alert allergic consumers but not a requirement. It is wise to choose products that you know or avoid using a new product until you have called the manufacturer to check if it is safe for you.

If the product is made in a different country (especially countries where allergies are less common), you have to be more careful. The common advice is to stick with products made in North America. Different countries have different food labelling standards. If there is a different flavour or variety of the same food that contains your allergen, and they look like they were made in the same place, it is worth investigating further to see if they were made with the same ingredients or in a different facility or country. Take the following as an example: You are allergic to peanuts and see that a regular box of cookies has no "may contain" statement on it. However, the smaller snack-size package with mini cookies declares, "may contain peanuts". It is definitely a good idea to call the company to get clarification on why there is a difference between the two packages of the same product brand.

As of August 4, 2012, a new set of food allergen labelling regulations was put into place in Canada. These regulations cover both pre-packaged food produced in Canada and pre-packaged food imported to Canada. The new regulations state that:

1.  While it is still necessary for foods to be listed in decreasing order of amount, some ingredients used in food products were previously exempt from declaration (such as components (part of a part) of margarine, or seasonings). If they are a priority allergen (see Chapter 2), these components must now be listed as well. For example, "mustard" would need to be shown if it is a component of "spices" and "milk" as an ingredient of margarine.[9]

2.  Ingredients that use scientific words for allergens must use clearer/common language in English and French. For example, "albumen" must show the word "egg."[10]

The new regulations apply to the list of "priority allergens" that have been identified as most likely to cause serious allergic reactions for Canadians. Priority allergens now include peanut, tree nuts (almonds, Brazil nuts, cashews, hazelnuts, macadamia nuts, pecans, pine nuts, pistachios, walnuts), milk, egg, seafood (fish, crustaceans, shellfish), soy, wheat, sesame seed, mustard, and sulphite. Companies have the option to either list the allergens on the ingredient list, in common language in parentheses following the un-common word or list them in a separate "contains" statement at the end of the ingredient list. If this option is used all of the allergens in the product must be listed in the "contain" statement. It is wise to remember that not all companies will use this option to provide allergen information therefore, you should

---

[9 10 11] Health Canada. *Food allergen labelling.* http://www.hc-sc.gc.ca/fn-an/label-etiquet/allergen/index-eng.php. Accessed: 16 January 2015.
[12] Health Canada. *Health Canada's Position on Gluten-Free Claims* http://www.hc-sc.gc.ca/fn-an/securit/allerg/cel-coe/gluten-position-eng.php. Accessed: 25 February, 2015

always read the entire ingredient list as well as the "contains" statement.

Health Canada has also included gluten sources and added sulphites to the new priority allergen list. This will increase food choices available to Canadians with food intolerances, Celiac disease[11] and sulphite reactions. Companies are now able to indicate that products are "gluten-free" if they unintentionally contain very small amounts of gluten [e.g. below 20 parts per million (ppm)].[12] However, it is important to remember that gluten free products may not be safe for someone who has a severe wheat allergy.

## Limiting the number of Precautionary Statements

There have been numerous and sometimes confusing terms used by manufacturers to alert allergic consumers of the possible presence of unintentional allergen in a product. To help consumers, Health Canada has encouraged manufacturers to use only one precautionary warning statement "may contain X" instead of the variety of phrases that you can find.[13] But remember, "may contain" statements are not required by law and companies can choose to use different phrases to say "may contain". *Although these claims are not part of the labelling law they must be truthful and not misleading.*

*Quick Tip - Companies can choose to put "free from" logos on their products to assist consumers in finding products that do not contain specific allergens. Although these logos are not part of the labelling laws the claims they make are held to the same standards as the precautionary statements and must be truthful and not misleading. There are many products that have a peanut-free symbol but do not indicate that they are also tree nut free. This is because they can*

---

[13] Health Canada. *Food allergen labelling.* http://www.hc-sc.gc.ca/fn-an/label-etiquet/allergen/index-eng.php. Accessed: 16 January 2015.

*scientifically test for the presence of peanuts in the products and on the processing equipment but cannot scientifically test for all of the tree nuts. A product can indicate that it is peanut free but also indicate that it "may contain" tree nuts or it might say that it contains tree nuts. This may seem confusing but technically it is correct as the product does not have peanuts. So it is important not to rely only on the "free from" symbol on the front of a package make sure you also read/check the ingredient list carefully.*

## What would you say? (Q&A)

*Caitlin F, Katelyn, Michelle*

**Have you ever had a reaction because you missed an ingredient?**

**Caitlin** - Yes, one time I had bought a package of curry mix that had "cream" as an ingredient. In retrospect, I could not believe it slipped past me when I was scanning the ingredients. However, I think I was just so focused on scanning for the usual words - milk, eggs, nuts, or peanuts.

**Katelyn** - I have never missed an ingredient or had a reaction because of it. I always make sure I read the labels of products I choose to consume. Recently, I have started calling the companies of products to inquire if there is any possibility of cross-contamination on their production lines.

**Michelle** - A long time ago, on Halloween, I was reading ingredients too fast because I was excited. I missed the clearly printed ingredient: peanuts. When I first took a bite, I realized that the chocolate seemed different and immediately stopped mid-bite. I spit out the treat, washed my mouth out, brushed my teeth, and told my mom. Thankfully, I had only touched the chocolate of the treat not the filling. So I didn't have a reaction. I was really lucky and, ever since then, I have always been really careful to read labels and even check with the company directly if I'm ever unsure.

**Do you eat products labeled "may contain"?**

**Caitlin -** I have had products that were labeled "may contain" before and have luckily never had a reaction.

**Katelyn -** I have eaten products labeled "may contain" in the past. Thankfully, I was lucky enough to not have a reaction. Gaining more knowledge about my allergies has given me a better grasp on risk analysis in certain situations. And I have come to the conclusion that it is simply not worth taking a risk with products I am unsure of. This doesn't mean that you have to deprive yourself! There are many companies that make products similar that adhere to allergy-safe standards. These companies are more than willing to provide you with all the information you need to make a logical decision.

**Kyle –** At one point I did. Once I had a severe reaction to a product labelled "may contain" and I will never touch them again.

**Michelle -** I have eaten products that are labeled "may contain" before, but have worked on avoiding them as I know it's not worth the risk. Lately, I find it's a lot easier to find alternatives. Having an allergy also makes it easy to turn down desserts and treats that I shouldn't be eating anyway.

**At what age did you start to read your own ingredient lists?**

**Caitlin -** I started to read my own ingredient labels around grade one. At this age, I could identify the words "milk, eggs, nuts, and peanuts." Of course my parents would read them with me at this age. But they believed it was never too early to get me to start with reading ingredients and building a routine of checking the label before I ate anything.

**Katelyn -** From a very young age, I learned to read my own ingredient labels. Let's just say I didn't have the best support group present at a young age. However, due to my independence, I did learn something from it! They didn't have the same labelling laws when I was younger. So I looked up alternative names for my allergens and made sure that there was nothing that could cause me to have an allergic reaction. By becoming familiar with these names (including ingredients in cosmetic products), I was able to determine that I had a passion for science and have started to build my career aspirations around it.

**Michelle** - My parents started to read labels with me as soon as I was capable of understanding what ingredient lists were in early elementary school.

**Sometimes we are in situations where others read ingredient lists for us. Do you trust others doing this for you?**

**Caitlin** - I generally trust close friends and family to read ingredient labels for me. However, I very often double-check the ingredients as well. I believe that having two sets of eyes scan the ingredients can help reduce any anxiety that I may have when trying a new food.

**Katelyn** - I only trust a small amount of people with reading ingredients for me. If I don't feel comfortable with the situation, then I ask if I can double-check for myself. It also helps, during the holidays for example, if you ask the host to keep the packages that the product was contained in.

**Michelle** - I will trust close family and some friends to check labels. Usually these are people who I have specifically taught to check labels the way I would. If someone else is insisting on reading the label for me, I sometimes find that it's awkward to ask to double-check. At parties and gatherings, I generally ask for the packages to be kept so I can look them over myself.

**What's the best AND worst part of reading ingredients for everything you eat?**

**Caitlin** - The worst part of reading ingredients is usually the fact that it is time-consuming. The best part of reading ingredients, however, is that it has made me much more aware of everything I eat. I believe I live a healthier lifestyle because of this.

**Katelyn** - The best part about reading an ingredient list for everything I eat is that I can also assess the nutritional information about the product. So I can also make good choices about my overall health. The worst part about reading an ingredient list on everything I eat is that it is time-consuming. But, in the end, it's worth it.

**Michelle** - I find it interesting to look at ingredients to see if it's something I could potentially make at home for myself. The worst part about reading ingredients is finding the original packaging. Some individually wrapped items have no labels because they're from a larger package that features the label.

To wrap it up...

As a teen with food allergies, you will become a master of label reading (if you aren't already). You can have much more peace of mind in knowing what exactly you are eating by:

1.  Recognizing the different names of your allergens
2.  Avoiding products with precautionary "may contain" warnings
3.  Calling companies for clarification
4.  Knowing when to trust others and not to be embarrassed to ask to double-check
5.  Recognizing how labelling laws are different in other countries

After all, eating food should be enjoyable. It's hard to appreciate a food when you're uncertain about its ingredients.

Summary Tips

1) Do not take a chance with precautionary (like "may contain") labels.

2. Do the "triple check" and read the ingredient list at the store, at home, and before you eat.

3. Always check the ingredient list because sometimes ingredients or manufacturing practices change.

# Section B

# Situations

# Chapter 6
## *High School and Allergies*

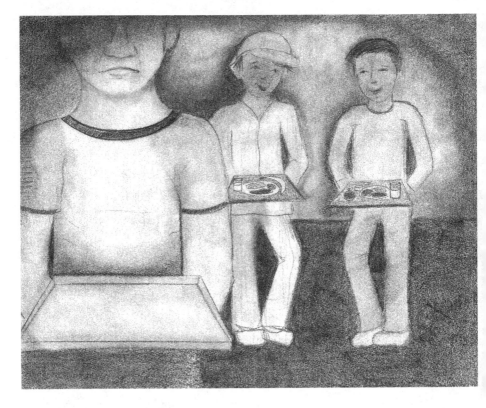

## Introduction

Remember how simple things were in elementary school? You had class with the same people, lunch was in the lunchroom, and homework never really took up too much of your time. There was so much structure like lining up after recess and the eagle-eye lunch monitors who made sure you washed your hands after you ate.

High school is a very different place from elementary school. Hundreds or even thousands of students are going every which way in this hyper-speed, mini-society filled with academics, arts, sports and, let's not forget, social drama! In the span of only one summer before high school, you are pushed into being more responsible for your grades, time management, decisions and, of course, your allergies. There's no magic formula to handle it all like a pro. But hearing how others have managed can definitely help.

## When things go right

### High School Non-Confidential, by Nicole

There were a few strategies that I used which made my transition to high school very easy. I had a few close friends who I had trained to use my auto-injector. In every class, I ensured that at least one person aside from me was trained, and comfortable, using my auto-injector in the event of an emergency. Even though high school has different classes with different teachers, I took the time to notify each of my teachers about my allergies. I carried my epinephrine in my purse and kept this with me at all times. I just didn't feel secure storing my auto-injector in my locker. How would anyone get to it in an emergency? My high school had a lot of extracurricular fundraisers and special events. I found that, if I joined committees, I could have more of a say in the planning process. This allowed me to contact venues and help create menus for things like semi-formal events, leadership camps, and the prom. Overall, using my voice and planning ahead really made high school an enjoyable time for me. I definitely didn't let my allergies stop me from doing the things I wanted to!

### Confidence Breeds Safety, by Michelle

Going through high school with an allergy can seem like a daunting task but, really, if you understand your allergy and know how to be safe, high school can be a breeze. I was careful to make sure I had knowledgeable friends who would stand up for me just in case I had to deal with someone who didn't understand. I also brought a lot of extra auto-injectors to school. I had one in my locker, just in case I forgot my belt one day, one in my lunch bag, and two on me at all times. In the beginning, I kept one in the office and left some with my teachers too. But that seemed unnecessary. So just keeping one in my locker, and two in my purse as I got older, was enough security. Whenever there were class parties or cooking classes, I always made an effort to make suggestions for alternative, safe foods that I could bring or others could easily find. Making yourself heard and being confident enough to explain the necessity of your safety are key when it comes to creating a safe environment for yourself.

*Quick Tip* - **The two-person rule:** *It is always a good idea to make sure that there are people around you who know about your allergies and who know what to do in an emergency situation (including how to use your auto-injector and where you keep it). These people can be friends, teachers, coaches or anyone else you trust.*

## When things go wrong

**Did I Hear You Right? By Nick**

When I was in grade 10, the relationship between my friends and my food allergy was odd at best. Personally, I am at risk for anaphylaxis to peanuts and tree nuts. My friends were aware that I wasn't allowed to eat certain foods. And they understood the consequences of eating those certain foods. Although this was great, their true understanding of how allergies worked was limited. This was clearly shown one day when a friend of mine wanted to perform a science experiment on me.

She asked what would happen if she stuck a peanut in my ear. I first laughed at the absurdity of the idea. But then I was horrified at her lack of understanding of the situation. Was she being serious? Was this a joke in poor taste? I certainly didn't find it funny. Trying my best not to over react, I tried to explain the seriousness of the situation and how anaphylaxis actually works. By the end of our conversation, I felt that I had gotten through to her and handled the situation properly.

**Take Me Out of the Ball Game, by Karen**

In grade 9 I started playing on the rugby team at my high school. We were all getting pumped up for our first rugby game ever. It also happened to be student council elections at the time. At my high school, candidates like to give out free treats and candies in order to win your vote. Now that's a way to "sugar-coat" politics! I had always been aware of the possibility of cross-contamination and "may contain" statements on ingredient lists. But that day, when I was running down the hall to go out to the field, my friend stopped me and asked if I could grab a brownie for her. Since I was so distracted by the fact that I was about to play a game, I grabbed the brownie, took a nibble, and ran out. The next thing I knew, I started having a reaction during warm-up. My friends on the team noticed right away that something was wrong. To be honest, I was in denial because I really wanted to play in the game. But my friend started walking me over to my bag to get my auto-injector. Once I had it in my hand, all the practice of using my auto-injector came in to play. I knew it was the right decision to use it as soon as I possibly could. To this day, I always remember to be aware of what I am eating whenever I get my hands on any type of food, regardless of the situation that I am in.

*Quick Tip* - *Many high schools have specific allergy policies that are in-line with provincial or school district guidelines. Check your high school's website or ask your principal about the details that apply specifically to your school.*

**What would you say? (Q&A)**

*Emily Rose, Samantha, Sydney H.*

**Was it easy to transition from elementary school to high school? What was the hardest part?**

**Emily Rose** - I found it easy to handle my allergy in high school. My school is very aware of allergies and has great protocols in place. The biggest difference I noticed is that I was more independent with my allergy. My teachers in elementary school would noticeably try to make sure I was safe and reinforce that peanuts were not allowed at school. In my high school, people can bring peanuts. So it is my job to make sure I stay vigilant and safe.

**Samantha** - I found it was relatively easy because I tried to figure everything out in advance and be prepared for any situations that might come up in a new environment.

**Sydney H.** - Transitioning from elementary to high school was difficult for me because I developed my allergies at the end of grade eight. When I began high school, I was still figuring out the precautions that needed to be taken and how to be responsible for my health and safety. I didn't want to be different from my peers. So I was in denial about having allergies for a while. Now, in grade twelve, I have it all worked out. My friends and classmates are very supportive of the challenges I face as a result of my allergies. For me, the hardest part was adjusting to a new school's way of handling allergies.

## How many of your high school teachers know/knew about your allergies?

**Daniela** - I did not tell all of my teachers about my allergies. I always, however, made sure there were at least two people in each class who knew about my allergies and knew how to use my auto-injector (since I had classes with many of the same friends, this was very easy). I also always made sure to tell the coaches of sports teams, my band teacher who took us on trips, and any teachers responsible for field trips or outings about my allergies.

**Samantha** - All of my teachers know about my allergies. I have personally told them about it, and it also states on the attendance sheet which students have life-threatening allergies.

**Sydney H.** - At the beginning of every semester, I always give my new teachers a letter explaining my allergies and my medical emergency plan. I also speak to them after class on the first day to explain the severity and how they can help.

**Where did/do you carry your auto-injector when at elementary school? High school?**

**Emily Rose** - In elementary school, I carried my auto-injector on me in a little bag. In high school, I always have a purse or backpack. So it is in there.

**Samantha** - In elementary school, I had an auto-injector pouch where I kept mine in it. In high school, I keep it either in a purse or in my backpack. But I prefer my purse because it is on me at all times.

**Sydney H.** - In elementary school and high school, I always carried two auto-injectors in my bag and there was always a spare one in the school office. My teachers and friends were always aware of where my auto-injector was kept.

**What's the best piece of advice you would give to someone entering high school?**

**Sydney H.** - I would say just be yourself and never downplay your allergies to fit in. If people are not willing to accept you, and respect your safety, then they are not your friends!

**Samantha** - Make sure to plan ahead and talk to the principal about your allergies before the school year begins. Double-check that all of your teachers are trained how to use an auto-injector and that they know what to do in an emergency.

**Emily Rose** - I would tell them not to worry. I would also say to make sure that as many people know about your allergy as possible. The more people you make aware of your allergy, and the importance of keeping your allergen away from you, the less chance you have of encountering it.

**Were/are there safe foods for you in your high school cafeteria?**

**Emily Rose** - I don't purchase food from the cafeteria very often but, yes, everything the school sells is peanut-free.

**Samantha** - Yes, there are a couple of foods that are safe for me: pizza and french fries. I have asked them what they make on-site, and what is brought in. For the food that is made in the cafeteria, I know what the ingredients are and how it is made. However, I prefer to go with food that is sold in a package with proper labelling that I know is safe for me. Approaching it this way ensures that there is no chance for cross-contamination before it gets to me.

## To wrap it up...

The transition to high school is an exciting time full of new opportunities. Managing your allergies through the transition can be challenging at times. But, by ensuring that there are people around you who understand your situation, and being open about explaining your allergies to people you meet, the transition can be relatively seamless.

## Summary Tips

1) Give the updated proper health/emergency paperwork to the school every year.
2) Keep your auto-injector on you (backpack, purse or pocket) rather than leaving it in your locker.
3) Look out for yourself by asking about food in the cafeteria, washing your hands, and being aware of cross-contamination.

# Chapter 7
## *Parties*

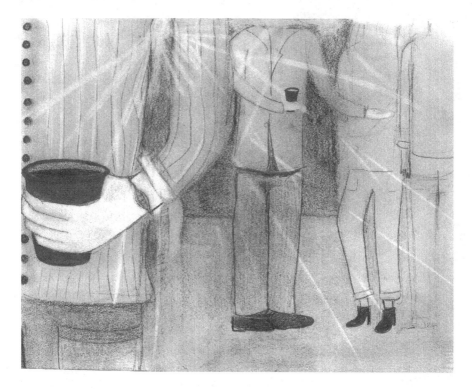

## Introduction

As a teenager, there will likely come a time when you will start to attend larger parties often involving alcohol (if you haven't already). Parties can be a lot of fun. Yet, they can sometimes include tricky situations when you've got allergies. For example, someone may offer you an unfamiliar drink, cups might be shared, people may pull out snacks that contain your allergen, and you may find that you are not entirely sober while you are trying to figure out how to handle these situations.

When you're facing any new or uncertain situation, it is always important to have a plan for how you will manage your allergies. At a party, figure out things like where you will put your auto-injector, who will be there that knows about your allergies, what you will be drinking, and what you will do if you get into an uncomfortable situation. Thinking through these things ahead of time will allow you to be safe and ready to have fun!

## When things go right

### Peanut Proofing the Party, by Dylan

When I was 16, I went to a New Year's Eve party at the house of a friend that I wasn't really close with. I knew him from a few classes at school. I tried to mention my severe peanut and tree nut allergies to him in the halls between classes. But, I never got the chance and I didn't have any of his contact information. So I was forced to go to the party a little earlier than I had originally planned. When I arrived, there were only a few people there. So I took the opportunity to scan the scene for the snack area. And what do I see? There was a plate full of all kinds of nuts freshly placed on a table surrounded by nut-free snacks! It was like looking at a food trap. I acted quickly and told the host about the severity of my allergies. He then brought me to talk to his parents who luckily understood and quickly took away the nut platter. They went on to show me every other snack's ingredients just to make sure everything was safe. And they even listened to my instructions about how to use my auto-injector in the worst-case scenario! What could have been a night filled with paranoia and anxiety turned into a really fun night with great friends!

### When Your Allergen is also a Party Guest, by Daniela

This past year, I was at a rugby team house party after a tournament. I was with a great group of friends and having a really fun time. I then noticed something that concerned me. There was a large container of peanuts sitting on a side table. And someone had just opened them and started passing them around. I realized quickly and asked, politely but firmly, if they could be put away. One of my friends realized too and made sure they were gone and that I was okay. Luckily I had caught the potential incident in time. For the rest of the night, however, I was extra vigilant in terms of making sure I didn't share any drinks or cups. It was a good reminder about how it's necessary to be aware of your surroundings and unafraid of standing up for yourself.

*Quick Tip* - *Get in touch with the party host in advance to find out what foods might be served. Offer suggestions or be willing to contribute safe snacks for the party.*

## When things go wrong

### This Party is Nuts! By Nicole

In the summer, I went to an outdoor barbeque party. The night got off to a really good start and I was having a lot of fun. As usual, I made sure that I ate a safe meal before the party to ensure that I wouldn't go hungry. I find that this always helps to alleviate the stress of finding something safe to eat when I am a guest in someone else's home. About an hour or so into the party, the host pulled out a gigantic, industrial-sized garbage bag filled with peanuts! The next thing I knew, *everyone* was eating them! I even saw people trying to throw nuts into each other's mouths! I immediately called my parents and had them come pick me up. I was disappointed that I couldn't stay at the party longer. However, I did not feel comfortable. In the end, it just wasn't worth it.

### Stop, Don't Shoot! By Caiti

A few summers ago, I was at a bachelorette party for a friend at her cottage. I brought my own beverages and food since I had read the labels ahead of time and knew that they were safe. As the night went on, I may have let my guard down a little. One of the bridesmaids, whom I had never met, was handing out Jello shots. I was offered one and, when I asked her what was in them, she simply replied "just Jello and alcohol." I asked to read the ingredients of both of them and, after discovering that they did not contain any of my allergens, I had one. A few minutes later, the girl had announced that she had also lined the containers with butter so that the Jello would "slip out easier." I am allergic to milk, and I immediately felt my throat getting itchy and I started getting hives. I took the auto-injector and had someone drive me to the hospital immediately. Thankfully, the reaction was not as severe as I had feared. I may not have even needed the auto-injector. However, I was really glad that I erred on the side of caution and took the epinephrine. After this experience, I learned that I should stick to having my own food and drinks at parties. I was thinking clearly. But others might not have been.

*Quick Tip* - Common allergens can sometimes be an ingredient in certain alcohols. Be sure to know what is safe for you to eat AND drink before you party. Don't be afraid to ask questions to the bartender or host about ingredients.

## What would you say? (Q&A)
*Hannah, Karen, and Nick*

**What do you do with your auto-injector at parties?**

**Hannah** - My auto-injector is always in my purse and I always bring my purse with me wherever I go. I don't just leave it at the door or with my coat, either. I'm always wearing it on me or have it with me.

**Karen** - I do not like to carry purses or clutches with me whenever I go out. So, sometimes, if I have to carry a purse, I will. But I normally carry it in my pocket. I recently got a new auto-injector that fits perfectly in my back pocket. It was the best allergy-related decision I've recently made!

**Nick** - I personally have my auto-injector in a pocket or somewhere else on my person at all times when partying.

**Do you share cups with other people?**

**Hannah** - Whether I'm on the bench during a sports game or at a party, I never share cups. You never know if someone has eaten your allergen earlier in the day. And the chance of cross-contamination is too great of a risk for me. I just don't feel comfortable doing it.

**Karen** - Yes, I share cups with people. I understand that it is not the safest decision. However, I like to think that I am smart about it. The only time I share cups with anybody is if I am friends with them and if I ask them what they have eaten during the day. I only ever do this at small gatherings with my close friends. And when I ask them what they've eaten, they almost always sit back and really think about what they've eaten. And, when they realize that they ate something containing my allergen, they say "Oh, never mind. You can't have that."

**Nick** - Never. It is impossible to track down what was in that cup or what the other person was eating. As a general rule, don't share drinks!

**What do you do if someone offers you a drink or a sip of their drink?**

**Hannah** - If someone offers me a drink, or asks to share mine, I simply say "Sorry, I can't. I have allergies." I've never had one person ask me for a greater explanation than that. Everyone just accepts it as fact.

**Nick** - Considering that this is an allergy safety hazard, and a general safety hazard, I would probably just say "No thanks" and that would be it.

**Karen** - Unless I see them pour a drink into a brand new cup straight from an unopened bottle, I normally do not take anything from anyone. Usually, if it's somebody I don't really know, then I just politely decline.

**Have you ever felt unsafe at a party because of your allergies?**

**Hannah** - If I go to a party, I try to eat before I go. And I will either bring my own drink or get a drink when I get there and keep it to myself the entire night. This way, I never feel unsafe.

**Nick** – Sometimes. But I generally don't eat food at a party. I normally eat before I go or I eat afterward.

**Karen** - Yes, absolutely. Whenever I go to party that actually has food being served, a lot of the time there is a mixture of nuts on display in multiple bowls all over the room. I always feel uncomfortable being surrounded by my allergens when I cannot control it. If it is a party being thrown by a friend, I will ask to see if they can be put away—which has happened and allows me to enjoy the party. Sometimes, though, I just leave because it's not worth the risk of sticking around and possibly having a reaction.

**Have you ever done something in advance of a party to make sure you're safe?**

**Hannah** - I always make sure that at least one friend at the party with me is aware of the risks associated with partying and having allergies. It's always good to have someone there for you in case things go wrong.

**Karen** - Whenever my friends and I have dinner parties, I always make a point of reminding them about my allergies in the hope that they remember when they're cooking. It never hurts to remind people, even those who are super close to you, about your allergies.

**Nick** – I always make sure I have my auto-injector with me. I also always have my wallet with my health card, a cell phone, and a friend that I trust.

**Have you ever heard of alcohol that contains your allergen?**

**Hannah** - I was shocked to learn that there are some alcohols that can contain allergens. Although they're not the most common, some are used for cooking and some rum is made with nuts! It's important to know what drinks you can and cannot have.

**Nick** – Yes, but I was only fourteen at the time. So it didn't mean much to me back then. However, as a twenty-year-old now, it is much more important to know. When you drink you may become inebriated and be unable to make well-thought-out decisions. So it is really important to understand what drinks are unsafe and stick with what you know is okay.

**Karen** - Yes, and I was happy to have figured that out before getting into partying with my friends. I now look up ingredients of alcohols that I've never tried before just to be on the safe side.

To wrap it up...

As a teen with food allergies, it is important to realize that you don't have to miss out on normal teenage experiences like going to parties. That being said, parties can be one of the more dangerous settings for those of us with allergies because, especially when alcohol is involved, people are often not making the best decisions and situations can get out of hand quickly.

The most essential thing you can do to keep yourself safe at a party is to ensure that you have at least one auto-injector *on your person*. While it is great to have one in your purse, or in your jacket at the door, it can easily get buried under a messy pile of coats and be very difficult to find if you are having a reaction. At some parties, there is even a chance that a purse or jacket could be stolen. To be safe, then, it is a really good idea to bring two auto-injectors. Furthermore, it is important that you tell your friends where your auto-injector is and to ensure that they know what to do if you have a reaction.

Aside from making sure you are well prepared with your auto-injector, know what (or if) you'll be drinking and what you would do in situations where drinks or cups are being shared. Doing research about which types of alcohol contain your allergen is key. And bring your own alcohol so you know it is safe. If drinks are being shared, be aware that either the drink may contain your allergen or whoever is offering the drink may have consumed your allergen(s) at some point throughout the day. Often, it is better to be safe and politely decline unless you are sure that the drink is safe and the person has not consumed your allergen(s). Sharing cups can also be dangerous. It is safest to find (or bring) clean cups or at least wash the cups before you use them.

If food is being served at a party, talk to the host before it is brought out to make sure that there's nothing that will put you in danger. However, unexpected situations do happen and, suddenly, there may be food brought out that you are very allergic to. In these types of situations, stay calm and politely, but firmly, explain that the food needs to be put away or moved to another room. Or, if you feel it is out of your control, it might be best to call it a night.

Finally, it's necessary to recognize that, if you have been drinking, you may not be able to make appropriate judgment calls about what is "safe." Put simply, you are more likely to take risks if alcohol is involved. Compromising your safety by drinking too much is never a good idea. And we hope that, by reading this chapter, you've realized some of the risks associated with going out to parties. But we also hope that you'll be able to incorporate our tips and advice so that you can enjoy going to parties safely.

## Summary Tips

1) Get in touch with the party host in advance and let them know about your allergies.
2) Remember that common allergens can be found in alcohol.
3) Always bring your auto-injector with you when going to a party.

# Chapter 8
## *Travelling*

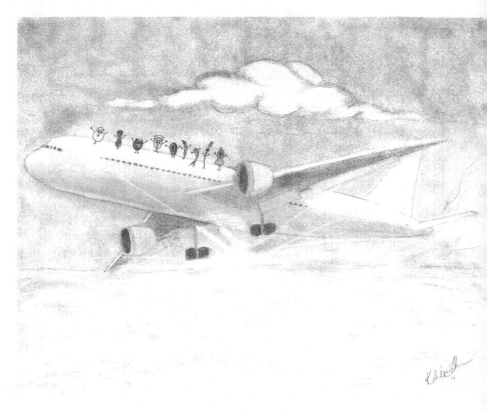

## Introduction

Travelling is often one of the most challenging situations you'll face when you have allergies. In this chapter, you will find out that, when you plan ahead, do your research, and get creative, it is possible to go almost anywhere.

There are definitely some places that are easier to visit than others. Things get more difficult if there is a language barrier, if the cuisine in the area often uses your allergen(s), or if the place is somewhere where allergies are much less common. However, even in the more difficult places, it is still possible to have an enjoyable trip if you're vigilant and well prepared.

**Breaking Down Language Barriers, by Lindsay**

When I was in high school, I took my first big trip without my family. I travelled to 6 different countries in Europe over the course of 6 weeks as I participated in a study-abroad program. Only one of the countries I travelled to had English as their primary language. I was, therefore, quite fearful about not being able to properly communicate with others about my allergies. Before I went on my trip, I spoke to my allergist about any specific locations I was going to that commonly serve foods containing my allergens. I also found a company on the Internet that creates laminated translation cards in many different languages. They contain messages explaining what your allergies are, asking for the nearest hospital, and with pictures of your allergens. While on my trip, these cards were very helpful as we frequently ate out at restaurants. I was able to feel comfortable and confident that the staff knew and understood my allergies. I was reaction-free on my trip and would recommend getting translation cards to anyone travelling somewhere with languages that are foreign to you!

Being on a trip with such a big group of people, I also found that it was important to speak up about my allergies and make sure that everyone was aware of my dietary restrictions. One day our teachers had booked a group lunch at a Chinese restaurant. They told me that they had spoken to the staff about my allergies. When we sat down, the first dish that was brought out had peanuts in it. Before I even realized this, someone in my group quickly told me to not eat the food. It was really great to see that others were so proactive about my allergies. I was accompanied by a friend to go eat at a different restaurant and avoided any potential risk of coming into contact with my allergen.

**Call Ahead Before You're Fed, by Arianne**

I have always been wary of eating sweets of any kind. Since my allergies to peanuts and nuts are very severe, and people tend to like nuts in sweets, they've always been a 'no- go'. A few years ago,

I had the opportunity to travel to Walt Disney World in Orlando, Florida. If you've ever been to Disney, you know that Mickey Bars are abundant in every park, resort, store, and on every corner! These delectable little treats are vanilla ice cream covered in dark chocolate. Given my allergies, I told myself that I wouldn't even look at them when I arrived. But my curiosity got the best of me and I did some research. I got in contact with the company who made them and it turns out that I was not the first person to inquire. I was told with the utmost confidence that they had not been made on a line or come into any contact with peanuts or nuts. Taking the time to look into something before my vacation allowed me to relax and enjoy the smallest thing like ice cream on a hot day. It is always important to be cautious and curious. Taking the right steps to determine if you can have something is rewarding because it gives you more insights into your surroundings and allows you to enjoy the little things in life with ease.

*Quick Tip - Some countries have different variations on recipes we think are familiar. They may add common allergens for different textures of flavours. Never make assumptions with a food that might usually be safe at home.*

## When things go wrong

**Cake Surprise, by Sydney P.**
While vacationing in Hawaii several years ago, I had the unfortunate outcome of an allergic reaction. I was having dinner with friends at a hotel restaurant. I had done my homework and called ahead to ensure that they could accommodate my food allergies to peanuts and tree nuts. Since there was no language barrier, I assumed that the kitchen staff understood my condition. My main course went by without incident and my anxiety had almost dissipated. I thought I was now in the clear. As we were getting ready to pay, the waiter arrived with a steaming lava cake in hand for my friend's birthday. While my friends started to dig in, I stood up, went to talk with the waiter, and inquired about the

ingredients. A few minutes later he returned from the kitchen with a smile. He declared that the chef had made the cake from scratch and that there was not a single nut inside. I felt slightly uncomfortable. But I decided to try some to join in the fun.

To make a long story short, I had an allergic reaction. I was well-equipped with my auto-injector and the hotel staff was quick to call an ambulance. The following day, after a not so exciting visit to the local emergency department, I returned to the restaurant to figure out what had happened. As it turns out, the chef was correct. The cake didn't have any nuts in it. But the waiter forgot to check the ingredients in the ice cream piled on top of the cake. I learned that macadamia nuts are a staple in Hawaiian cuisine. I learned many things from this experience: 1) If you have any doubt, whatsoever, don't risk it; 2) Always travel equipped with travel insurance; and, lastly, 3) Don't be embarrassed to ask to speak directly with the chef!

**Opened Eyes on the Open Water, by Talia**

Last summer, my parents and I went on a cruise around Italy. Every evening we would have dinner in the ship's dining room. When we booked the trip a few months prior, we informed the staff about my food allergies. The staff was very accommodating and assured me that there was a special section of the kitchen where "special orders" were prepared. They assured me that there would be no contamination with any of my allergens. The head chef even met with me to ask me what kind of food I liked!

One night, for dessert, we got chocolate cake. I asked the waiter if there were any nuts in the cake, just to be sure. He told me that there weren't. I had eaten quite a bit of the cake when I noticed little decorations on the cake. I asked my mother if they were edible. She paused, and then told me to put my fork down. It turns out that they were made of marzipan, which contains almonds (one of my allergens). This incident was a rude wake-up call. No matter how safe I might have felt or how well-intentioned someone might have been, the reality is that people make mistakes.

For every night after this experience, I made sure that the waiter double-checked everything that came out of the kitchen. I chose simple meals where I could see most of the ingredients and I skipped any chocolaty dessert from then on. My advice to anyone with food allergies is to, first and foremost, know your allergens and where they can hide. Making yourself informed and being vigilant are crucial because, in the end, no one is responsible for your health but you.

*Quick Tip* - *Consider making a food allergy "cheat sheet" for the place you're visiting. Write down translations of your allergens, foods to avoid, the local emergency numbers, and your own emergency contact information in case you need help.*

## What would you say? (Q&A)
*Daniela, Emily Rose, Giulia, Stephanie*

**Does airline travel make you nervous? Do you notify airlines ahead of time?**

**Emily Rose** - No I am not nervous to travel on an airline. I always call ahead to notify them. As well, when I get on the plane, I tell the flight attendants. They usually handle it very well and are helpful.

**Giulia** - I have never notified airlines ahead of time regarding my allergies. I usually notify the airline staff upon entering the plane and they have sometimes designated a 'safety zone' for me where the people three rows ahead, to the side, and behind me are asked not to eat my allergen. I have never had a bad experience on a plane and I, therefore, tend not to get nervous.

**Stephanie** - I am nervous when I fly because, if I have an allergic reaction, I want to make sure that I am prepared. I always carry my auto-injector, inform the airline in advance, pack my own food, and inform the flight attendants about my allergies. They are usually more than willing to accommodate me.

**Where is the most exotic place you have been with your allergies?**

**Daniela -** I went to Mexico for a conference while I was in middle school. It was tricky because I only knew a few phrases of Spanish and allergies did not seem common where I was. Since I was only gone for six days, I was able to bring some of my own food and I managed to find some basic food that I could eat while I was there.

**Giulia -** I have been to Costa Rica twice. I was initially anxious about travelling to such an exotic place with my allergies. But I found that they cooked very plainly. The most exotic dish I had was rice and beans!

**Stephanie -** I travelled throughout Poland with my allergies! I speak the language and stayed with family. So it was a fantastic experience where I could eat the food. It was just like being at home!

**What do you do in situations where there is a language barrier?**

**Giulia -** Before leaving for any exotic place, I write down the translations of my allergens on a piece of paper and practice how to say the information I may need to explain to someone on my trip. You always need to ensure that there are no misunderstandings when your allergies are involved!

**Stephanie -** I brought cards with my allergies written on them to various countries and showed them to the staff at restaurants and bakeries to ensure that they understood my allergies. I translated, "I am allergic to..." with an online translator.

**Planes, trains, ships or automobiles – what's the toughest form of travel with allergies?**

**Emily Rose -** I would say planes. This is because planes sometimes sell peanuts. So I have to be extra careful. I always clean the area where I will be sitting and put a towel down just in case the person before me ate peanuts.

**Giulia** - I am very hesitant to travel on a boat with my allergies. The enclosed space and travelling in the open water without access to any sort of hospital makes me very anxious.

**Stephanie** - Planes might be the toughest because you do not know who you will be sitting beside and you cannot change your seat very easily. I have been a little too close for comfort to people eating foods I am allergic to on planes before.

### How many auto-injectors do you take with you when travelling?

**Emily Rose** - It depends on what method of transport I will be taking. In a plane, I take six auto-injectors. So I will have a lot of spares if I have a reaction. If I am travelling by bus or car I take three - two to carry on me and one extra just in case.

**Giulia** - It is a minimum of 4 for me. You need to bring at least 2 just in case you have a biphasic reaction (i.e. a reaction that comes back after the initial reaction). You always need to bring backups just in case something was to happen!

**Stephanie** - I take, at the very least, two auto-injectors with me to be safe!

### What safe food do you bring with you when travelling?

**Emily Rose** - I bring a lot of packaged food. Packaged snacks are always good. Instant noodles can also come in handy.

**Giulia** - I always bring safe protein bars wherever I go. If you can't eat something, and you're hungry, a protein bar will give you the efficient nutrition needed to keep going!

**Stephanie** - I carry allergen-free granola bars, sandwiches, bagels, cheese, homemade cookies, dried fruit, and fresh fruit! Some of this will last for longer into my trip. But other foods need to be eaten sooner. It is important to be prepared with extra food in case your flight is delayed.

**At what age did you first travel without your parents?**

**Daniela** – I went to Mexico at age 12 without my parents.

**Emily Rose** - I'm looking forward to this someday!

**Giulia** - I'm turning 21 this year and hope to go on my first trip overseas without my parents!

**Stephanie** - I went on my first flight alone at the age of 19.


## To wrap it up...

From reading this book so far, you may have gathered that allergies shouldn't stop you from doing anything as long as you take the proper precautions. Plan ahead and be vigilant. Yes, this includes when you are travelling!

Doing your research ahead of time, informing others about your allergies, and bringing enough epinephrine are all essential to having a safe journey. Calling airlines ahead of time may be something you choose to do, especially for longer flights, to ensure that you stay safe while in the air.

It is also important to realize that, if there is a place that you really want to visit, your allergies shouldn't hold you back. If there is a language barrier, it will be more difficult. But, by bringing translation cards and learning a few phrases in the language, you will be able to communicate your allergies. If you are travelling to a place where your allergen(s) are a staple in the local cuisine, it will be important to find simple foods that you know are safe. And it may be useful to bring some of your own food. If you do your research, get creative, and stay determined, you will find a way to make it work!

## Summary Tips

1) Plan ahead and look into local cuisine, emergency numbers, and travel insurance.
2) Bring extra auto-injectors and safe snack food with you, especially for a plane. Remember that not all countries have the same auto-injectors as in Canada and some countries don't have epinephrine auto-injectors at all.
3) Consider getting your allergies translated for international travel.

# Chapter 9
*Dining Out*

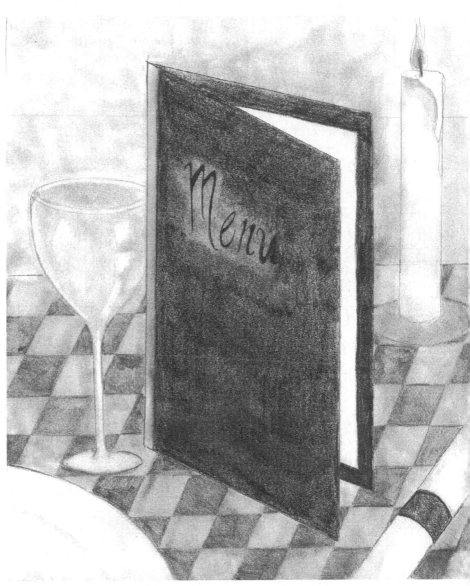

## Introduction

When you were a kid, your mom or dad probably pulled the waiter aside, explained your allergies, and made sure you got a safe meal. You may not have realized it, but they probably took the worrying off of your plate: no pun intended. But now, as a teen, you can probably think of many situations where you wouldn't want a parent tagging along. Maybe you're going for a team dinner, grabbing a slice of pizza with friends, or even going on a date. Imagine if your mom came with you on a first date to make sure your food was safe—talk about a third wheel! Learning how to advocate for yourself while you're dining out will allow you to enjoy a lot of fun situations as a teen and young adult.

Dining out with allergies can be tricky. But there are a number of things you can do to make it an enjoyable experience. Calling restaurants ahead of time, speaking to wait staff, talking to a chef or manager, and explaining the severity of your allergy/allergies, including the risks of cross-contamination, are a few skills that will help you have a great time while enjoying your meal with some peace of mind.

## When things go right

**At Your Service, by Nicole**
One summer day, I was walking downtown with my friend. We had been shopping all day and were famished! We noticed that a brand new restaurant was open. Despite having some of my allergens on the menu, we still decided to eat there. I am allergic to all seafood and I've found that most restaurants do have seafood somewhere on their menu. However, by speaking to the wait staff and manager, I can usually find a safe option that has minimal risk of cross-contamination. I mentioned my allergens to the waiter. Immediately, the manager came over and began to offer some options that would be safe for me. If that wasn't enough, the manager then went back to speak to the kitchen staff. The next thing I knew, one of the cooks came out and spoke to me about the dish I ordered! I was so impressed! I felt very secure and was grateful that all staff members at this restaurant were knowledgeable and willing to assist me in finding a safe option to eat. My meal was delicious and I left with a huge smile on my face!

**Opening up Restaurant Doors, by Caiti**

Throughout high school, I tended to avoid dining out. I would never eat the cafeteria food at school or order anything at a restaurant. I would bring safe lunches and dinners everywhere I went and I stayed on the lookout for a microwave to heat up my food. I just didn't feel comfortable dining out at all.

As I got older, I started facing another challenge—dating. I would always try to suggest options that didn't involve food whenever I was asked to go on a date. Whether it was golfing, going to the movies, or watching a hockey game, I always made sure that I would have a huge lunch to tide myself over. I did not want my allergies to stop me from having fun. So this compromise was okay.

Then I met my current boyfriend who goes above and beyond when it comes to my allergies. Early in our relationship, we had a lot of "dining-in" nights where we would cook together and he would learn to read ingredients thoroughly, wash his hands, and pay attention to avoiding cross-contamination. As time went on, he started researching restaurants that incorporate protocols that decrease the risk of exposure to allergens for allergic customers such as "allergy menus" and staff training. He then took me to one of the restaurants he had researched on a surprise anniversary date. He had called ahead to ask for a reservation and request that a manager be available for us to speak to regarding our allergies. When we arrived, I admit, I was a bit hesitant. However, the staff was extremely friendly and assured me that they've had many customers with similar dietary restrictions and that we were in good hands. We ordered our food and had a beautiful, delicious meal with no problems. I was so thrilled with the experience! Since then, we go out at least once a month to a restaurant from this chain and I am feeling more and more comfortable every time I dine out.

*Quick Tip* - *Calling a restaurant ahead of time or checking their website to see what they can do to accommodate your allergies are great ways to ensure that you'll be able to get a safe meal - especially when it is your first time going to a restaurant.*

**Not Confident about Over-Confidence, by Hannah**

I was recently vacationing. I went to a restaurant where the waiter seemed to be taking my allergies seriously. I didn't order anything that was risky for containing nuts. But I told the waiter about my allergies and asked him to tell the kitchen. He seemed a little too confident in his ability to know the exact ingredients of every item on the menu. When it came time for dessert, I decided to really test his knowledge. I had read over the dessert menu and knew that the key lime pie was made with a crust that had tree nuts in it—one of my allergens. I asked if any of the desserts were safe for me to eat. He said they were all fine and all delicious. In fact, the key lime was his favourite! I was shocked, upset, and obviously did not order any dessert. Sometimes, it's not enough to trust the wait staff. You need to be careful, observant, and extra vigilant when it comes to desserts. This experience reminded me to always keep my guard up and watch out for my allergens!

**After Dinner Surprise, by Erika**

A few years ago, my parents had flown across the country to visit me after I moved to the west coast. I had been with my boyfriend for 6 months. It was time that they met him. My parents took us out for dinner and I was very careful when ordering my meal. The server paid very close attention to make sure everything would be as safe as possible for me. I was being as responsible as I could be. Well, dessert came around, and I could not have any of the cakes or pies. So I decided to order a fancy coffee. As it turned out, the coffee that I ordered had an almond-based liqueur in it. I had missed that when I ordered the special coffee and had a slip-up. A few minutes later I started feeling sick and, by the time I had been dropped off at home, the symptoms were getting worse and worse. I then used my auto-injector and went to the hospital where soon the reaction was under control.

You can try to be as responsible as possible but, sometimes, we miss things. When things go wrong it is extremely important to act responsibly. What I learned from this situation was to take my epinephrine auto-injector right away and take responsibility for missing an unsafe ingredient in my coffee. That was the "meet the parents" night for my boyfriend. It was quite an eventful one!

*Quick Tip - Asking specific questions about the ingredients in whatever you're ordering can be really helpful in ensuring that the waiter understands the severity of your allergies. This helps give you peace of mind that there aren't any surprise allergens present. However, keep in mind that, even when we try our best to reduce the risks, accidents can still happen.*

## What would you say? (Q&A)
*Caitlyn P, Giulia, and Mathew*

**What is your little spiel that you give to the server at a restaurant?**

**Caitlyn** – I typically say something like: "I just wanted to let you know that I have severe food allergies. I am allergic to wheat, eggs, and nuts. So my food cannot contain or come in contact with any of these items. I was looking at your (insert menu item here). Would that contain any of these foods or do you have any other safe options on your menu?"

After inquiring about a specific menu item, or asking what allergen-free options are available, waiters tend to be very good about inquiring and talking to the kitchen and the chef. If they give you a generic reply such as "Oh, yeah that item is fine," don't be afraid to specifically ask them to go and verify with the kitchen for you or ask if you can speak to the chef or manager. It is important, even if the specific item you are ordering does not contain an allergen, that the area and tools used to prepare your meal are also free of cross-contamination.

**Giulia** - My little spiel goes a little like this: "Hi. I just want to inform you that I have a severe and life- threatening allergy to... Are there any accommodations you can make for me? I was also looking at this item on the menu and I wanted to know if it is safe for me."

**Mathew** – I find it depends on the situation. If I am in a rush, I will say: "I have a nut allergy. What would you recommend as being a safe choice? Something simple please..." If I have more time, and want to select something off of the menu, I say: "I have a nut allergy and was looking at the (insert dish here). Can you deal with allergies/have you dealt with them before? Can you speak with the kitchen staff?"

**Do you usually talk to the chef as well? The manager?**

**Caitlyn** - I will admit, I do not always talk to the manager or chef if the waiter or waitress is diligent at maintaining open communication between the kitchen and myself. I do find that, quite commonly, without even asking, the chef or manager will come over and meet with me to discuss what safe food options are available. This is always extra reassuring and shows that the restaurant is willing to take the extra steps to be allergy- friendly.

**Giulia** - Most of the time, my waiter or waitress informs me that they will be getting the manager to talk to me because they are more knowledgeable about dealing with allergy accommodations. I have never felt the need to also talk to the chef. Most restaurants that I've been to are pretty knowledgeable about the possibility of a customer having allergies and they take allergies seriously.

**Mathew** - I never ask to speak to the manager or chef. But this is definitely a good precaution to take. I have found that I can effectively communicate my issue to the waiter or waitress. It seems to me that allergies are becoming more common and, because of this, the staff's knowledge can be nearly as good as the manager's (although not always) through many experiences with diners who have food allergies.

**Is it ever a little bit awkward to have to explain your allergies? Any tips for making it less awkward?**

**Caitlyn** - I like to consider myself pretty comfortable when it comes to talking about my allergies. But my confidence has definitely grown over time. I find that there is a balance between trying to convey the seriousness of your allergies to wait staff and trying not to overwhelm them. I find it best to stay positive and confident when explaining your allergies. But don't skimp on explaining the facts and stressing important information such as staying diligent about cross-contamination.

**Giulia** - For sure! Especially when you're with a date or your friends and they all take 5 seconds to order. You feel like you're sitting there forever explaining your allergies to the waiter or waitress. I find that, to make it less awkward, you need to be confident! Show that it doesn't bother you! Chances are that, if you're confident, you really put everyone else at ease around you.

**Mathew** - Although it is not awkward for me now, it definitely used to be. I used to not like being the centre of attention and I didn't feel comfortable when someone was focused on what I was telling them about myself. I have overcome that and I am now happy to tell people about my allergy. Everyone has their own way of telling others about their allergies. I try to be blunt or joke about it. I don't hesitate to tell the person about the commotion that might happen if I ingest the allergen. Sometimes people will ask me if it is okay if they eat the allergen around me. I tell them, with a smile, to just try to resist the urge to kiss me!

**Do you ever call a restaurant in advance? If so, what do you say?**

**Caitlyn** - I have found restaurants to be very helpful for the most part when I've called ahead of time. Once you are talking to the right person, generally, they are very cooperative and informative. They want your business and will work to make a safe eating experience for you.

**Giulia** - I have called a restaurant in advance before. You want to make sure that you're not walking into a restaurant that absolutely cannot make accommodations for your allergens.

**Mathew** - I often don't do this. But it is a good precaution to take. If I were to call, I would say "I have a nut allergy. Can you accommodate this?" Each person you speak to regarding your allergies is different in terms of culture and current knowledge of allergies and language. The level of care you take when you talk to them will always differ. I would engage them in a conversation and ask them things such as: "Have you dealt with this before and is there anything on the menu with (insert allergen)."

To wrap it up...

It's great to see examples of restaurants accommodating allergies and having specific allergy-safe policies in place so that we can eat comfortably and safely. However, it is important to realize that situations can go wrong when wait staff do not grasp the severity of the allergy before recommending food items. Or, sometimes, there can be surprise ingredients in presumably safe foods. Knowing how to take the necessary precautions is essential to ensuring that you have a safe and fun time eating out.

Explaining your allergies to the server is a great first step. If you are trying out a new restaurant, it may be worth calling ahead to check if they are able to accommodate your allergies. When talking to a server, you can often tell whether or not they "get it." Once you have told them your allergies, explain the risks of cross-contamination and indicate what you are hoping to eat. Many servers will respond by saying whether or not they think the food item will be okay and explain that they will relay the information back to the chef. Sometimes, however, a server may seem overconfident and say that everything is okay. They may brush off your allergies like they are no big deal, they may seem extra worried about everything or they may tell you that they can't guarantee anything. In these situations, especially, it is a good idea to ask to speak with the manager or the chef directly to ensure that your allergies are clearly understood by the person making your food.

At first, dining out without your parents can be a bit stressful or difficult. But, as you learn exactly what to tell the waiter, you figure out when you need to talk to a chef or manager. Dining out can be a lot of fun and an awesome experience!

## Summary Tips

1) Plan ahead by either calling the restaurant or looking on their website for allergy information.
2) Tell the wait staff about your allergies and ask for safe food options.
3) Be sure that the people you're eating with know that you have allergies and where you keep your auto-injector.

# Chapter 10
## *The Workplace*

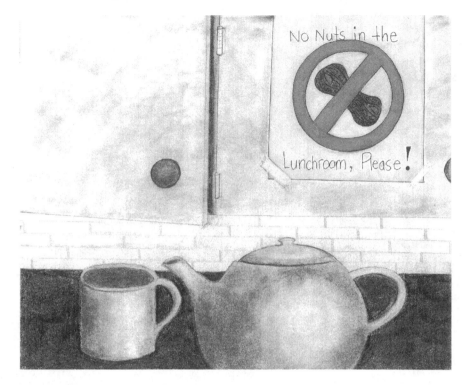

## Introduction

Whether you are getting your very first part-time job, working somewhere for the summer, or even starting a career, there will be a lot to think about when it comes to managing your allergies. You may be wondering: "When do I tell my employer about my allergies?" or "If I say I have allergies during an interview, will it lower my odds of getting a job?" or, maybe: "How will I make sure that I'm not in danger in the workplace?"

It is always important to be up front and honest about your allergies. Telling your employer is important. And telling co-workers can also be very helpful. The precautions you have to take will differ depending upon the nature of your work. If you are working in a restaurant, you may choose to work in a specific location or wear gloves when handling certain foods that contain your allergen. If your workplace orders meals, you may need to make arrangements so that there is something safe for you to eat. Remember, having a job is all about earning your livelihood, not risking it!

## When things go right

**Inform Others Early - Your Stomach Will Thank You Later, by Nick**
Last fall, I was lucky enough to land an internship with a start-up company in the city where my university is. The job itself was wonderful. It had many perks, including a free lunch every Friday. In my first week at the job, I wasn't too concerned about my food allergy. I was too busy fighting with my computer to install the correct software. However, on the Thursday before this lunch, I decided to ask our secretary what was for lunch that Friday. Chinese food with a lot of cashews and peanuts was her reply. Immediately I told her about my allergy and how serious it was. Luckily she understood and actually ordered pizza instead! For the rest of my internship, she consulted with me when picking food to make sure that I was safe in the work place.

**Bending over Backwards, by Dylan**
Last year, I worked at a physiotherapy and sports injuries clinic. Being a new person at a big job that I had worked so hard to get, I was a little nervous to bring up my severe nut allergy. After a few weeks, I finally told one of my co-workers about my allergy. Word spread like wildfire to the remaining seven employees. Before long, I had the owner asking me about the severity of my allergy and what kinds of foods she should avoid eating or bringing to the clinic! She even asked where I kept my auto-injector and made note of it in her little notebook. The administrative assistant at the clinic didn't understand the allergy at first. But she usually questioned everything she didn't understand. So I was soon confronted with hundreds of questions about my life! It was refreshing to see co-workers care as much as they all did. In fact, they even went so far as to declare the clinic "peanut/nut free"

with a sign in the window to let patients know too. This was by far the best experience I have ever had at a workplace and I strongly suggest speaking up to every co-worker about the severity of your allergy. Educate those around you and you may be surprised by how positive the outcome will be!"

*Quick Tip* - *Some workplaces may have never had an employee with your allergies before. Be sure to inform them and offer helpful suggestions about how they can make an allergy-safe workplace.*

## When things go wrong

**The Interview, by Erika**
I had interviewed for a position at a new company. I was worried that mentioning my severe food allergies might affect my chances of being hired. As such, I decided not to mention them. When hired, I told the HR person as well as my supervisor about my allergies and asked what accommodations they could make. At the time that I mentioned my allergies to them, I did not express how severe they were.

When a colleague left a box of nuts in the lobby for everyone to share, I got extremely scared. It meant that there were people eating nuts all around me and that the desk I work on would have nuts all over it. I tried to talk to them about my allergies again. Some colleagues and other staff did not really believe me that my allergies were so serious because I had downplayed them in the beginning. I did not want to be a burden or nuisance to others for whom nuts and peanuts were a staple in their diets. This led to me feeling guilty when colleagues would mention that they had to avoid bringing in foods they always used to eat. They noted that they were confused why they could not bring them in anymore. Looking back, I was wrong in the way that I had managed the entire situation of informing others about my allergies. I should have mentioned my food allergies in the interview process and informed of how serious they were. Had I done that, colleagues would have better understood the accommodations and might have been more likely to support and understand me.

**Camp Counsellor Conundrum, by Erika**

I worked at a summer camp and not all of my colleagues were fully aware of how serious my peanut and nut allergies were. I showed up for work one morning and started preparing to sign in children. Once the children had arrived, and we were ready to start the camp, I went to join the other camp counsellors and campers. And suddenly I freaked out. There was a huge bowl of trail mix on the picnic table and all the children were grabbing handfuls of nuts. I had no clue where the bowl of trail mix had come from. But I knew one thing. Having a dozen children under the age of 10 running around with hands that had touched tree nuts was really risky. They would be touching all the same equipment I would be touching. Plus the younger kids often tried to hug us or run up to us from behind. I was so overwhelmed and terrified that I failed to communicate to the camp leaders what was going on so they could remove the nuts. I went to the bathroom and cried. I was lucky that one of my friends, also a camp counsellor, understood my allergies and came to calm me down and re-assure me. He had the bowl taken away and all the kids had gone to wash their hands.

Looking back, there was no way for me to know that there was a bowl of trail mix out on the picnic table. However, I should have educated all the camp counsellors about the seriousness of my food allergies and perhaps they would have identified the threat sooner. I also should have said something before running away from the situation. I am, however, not upset about my reaction. I have learned from it and know that there are certain situations when our emotions take over and it is hard to control them. I was scared and I fled the situation. I was lucky to have a friend to help me. It is extremely important to speak-up about your allergies and educate those around you whether they are friends or colleagues.

*Quick Tip* - Informing co-workers will help ensure that you have a support network at the workplace and that others will know what's happening if you ever have an allergic reaction.

## What would you say? (Q&A)

*Caitlyn F. (Caiti), Erika, Sydney H.*

### Who do you explain your allergies to?

**Caiti** - I make an effort to tell everyone I can at my work place about my allergies. I also make sure that I train at least one person, whom I will be working with at all times, how to use my auto-injector.

**Erika** - In each place I have worked, I always tell my manager or supervisor about my allergies either when I am hired or on my first day of work. When I discuss my allergies, and the severity of them, I ask them what they believe would be the most appropriate way to inform my colleagues.

**Sydney H.** - I tell all my managers and supervisors about my allergies. I also make a point to tell my co-workers the first time I work with them. It's actually a good conversation starter and managers are always happy to know that you are responsible and honest.

### Do you explain that you have allergies before you are hired?

**Caiti** - I do make employers aware of my allergies. But I make sure I explain that it will not affect my performance at my job.

**Erika** - When I've believed it might be hard to keep my own environment safe, like in grocery stores that sell nuts in bulk, I have mentioned my allergies during interviews—before I am hired. There have been some jobs where I have not mentioned my allergies in the interview process. I thought my allergies might play a role in their decision to hire me. And, looking back, I wish I had told them.

**Sydney H.** - During a job interview, when the interviewer asks if I have any questions, I find that this is a good time to bring up my allergies and see what safety precautions will be taken. I have also asked whether any staff members are trained to give an auto-injector.

**Are there any places you would not want to work because of your allergies?**

**Caiti** - I would not feel comfortable working in the food industry (serving at a restaurant for example).

**Erika** - I would not want to work in a restaurant with foods that commonly have my allergens.

**Sydney H.** - I worked in the food industry for a while and ended up switching to retail because I found it too tricky with allergies. Clearing tables that contained my allergens just wasn't a safe decision for me to make. Now, in retail, I rarely come across allergens and feel a lot safer.

**Is the staff area/kitchen allergy safe?**

**Caiti -** Our staff area is fairly clean. However, things like the microwave, fridge, etc. are always a bit of a concern. I keep all of my food in my separate lunch bag. And I make sure that I wipe down any areas before I place my food anywhere.

**Erika** - I would always bring my own utensils and eat out of the plastic containers I brought from home. The kitchens were not safe. Employees continued to eat peanuts and nuts in the places I worked and, therefore, I always wiped down the table surface before I would sit down to eat my lunch. Or I would eat at my desk.

**Sydney H.** - Sometimes I do come across allergens at work. Specifically in the staff break room. But I always wipe down the table first and I am very aware of my surroundings.

**Where do you keep your auto-injector when you're on the job?**

**Caiti**- I always keep my auto-injector in my purse and I make sure that someone I am working with is aware of where it is kept.

**Erika** - In previous places of employment, I have always had my auto-injector on my desk, in plain sight, or in the desk drawer. In the second case, I have informed all of my colleagues where it can be easily found in an emergency.

**Do you take any precautions at work to avoid allergens?**

**Caiti** - Yes, I make sure to use sanitizing wipes to wipe down things like desks, phones, computer keyboards, etc. to avoid allergens. I also frequently use hand sanitizer.

**Erika** - When I worked in an office environment, I had my supervisor send an email out to all employees about my allergies and the severity of them. I made sure my desk and cubicle area was safe by asking my colleagues to avoid eating peanuts and nuts. And I informed others not to touch my phone or computer.

**Sydney H.** - The main precautions that I take are informing fellow employees and always remembering to bring my auto-injector to work!

To wrap it up...

The best attitude to take when managing your allergies in the workplace, or in any situation for that matter, is one that is proactive and responsible. It is important to explain your allergies early on to your employer so that they aren't caught off-guard later on when there is a tricky situation. Whether or not you talk about your allergies during the interview itself is up to you; however, if you are worried they will hinder your chances of getting the job, you can always explain that they will not affect your ability to work in any way.

Telling coworkers early on is also important. This is especially true if you need them to make accommodations for you (such as not bringing certain foods or washing their hands after handling an allergen). It is also a good idea to ensure that there are at least a few people who know where you keep your auto-injector and how to use it if you were to have a reaction. By taking the initiative to inform others, and making suggestions about how your employer and coworkers can help keep you safe, it will allow you to be comfortable and confident at work while proving your ability to be proactive.

## Summary Tips

1) Inform your boss or HR manager about your allergies either in your interview, or early on in your employment.
2) Let your co-workers know where you keep your auto-injector when working.
3) Never feel obligated to do a task that might put you in contact with your allergens. Talk to your boss regarding alternative tasks or accommodation.

# Chapter 11
## *College/University*

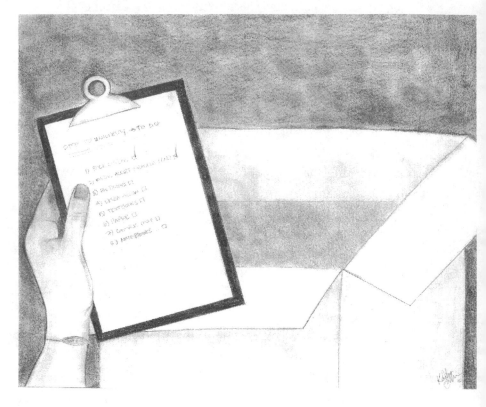

## Introduction

Heading off to college or university presents a wide array of new challenges. You will probably have questions like: "Should I have a roommate?", "Can I get a meal plan?", "Who should I talk to before I move in to residence?", and many others. Living in residence, meeting a whole bunch of people, eating in a cafeteria, living with friends, and cooking in a shared kitchen are some of the new situations that you will probably face.

In general, it is good to do a bit of research to find out what your school will offer in terms of living and eating accommodations. The situation varies between schools. But, generally, schools have many ways to help you out. And they may have set policies in place. By researching and preparing ahead of time, many teens and young adults have found the transition to college or university relatively seamless in terms of allergy management.

## When things go right

**Nothing to be Worried About, by Sydney P.**
I was a tad nervous when moving into residence for my first year of university. This was mainly because someone else was now in charge of cooking. I decided to e-mail the residence coordinator in July to give them plenty of notice that I suffer from severe food allergies to peanuts and tree nuts. I woke up the following morning to find a wonderful e-mail waiting for me in my inbox. I was being offered a single room to reduce the risk of being exposed to allergens in residence. And I was scheduled to meet with the head chef of food services on my move-in day to discuss how they could help accommodate me. I was overjoyed! While I was organizing my room on move-in day, in September, the residence coordinator herself came to meet me and she introduced my parents and me to the head chef in her office. He explained the various precautions they had in place to make eating safe. And they gave me his e-mail and phone number in case I had any more questions. To top it all off, the residence coordinator showed me around the cafeteria and explained what to watch out for. We finished the day by all eating dinner together. I could not have been more pleased with the way the residence staff handled my food allergies. I was able to go that entire school year reaction-free!

**A Smooth Transition, by Caitlyn**
When I was first thinking about going to university, I always thought that it would be cool to have a roommate. Well, wouldn't you know, lucky me, I didn't get just one roommate, I got TWO. I ended up being placed in a triple room. That's right folks. It was three girls surviving in one room for an entire school year! When I found out who my roommates were in the summer, I contacted both via e-mail right away to introduce myself. After establishing

who we were, I informed them both about my allergies and the seriousness of my peanut allergy. I was fortunate that both of them were very understanding about how serious it was. And they offered to not bring any peanuts into our room. Moving into residence was a hectic and exciting time and I was meeting a lot of new people. When I met my residence don, I told him about my allergies and the seriousness of them. By doing this, he was able to remind everyone on the floor as he met them that day that we had a floor member with life-threatening allergies.

On the same day that I moved into residence, I met both cafeteria chefs on campus so they would know me and know about my allergies. It was there that I found out that they had specially prepared allergy-friendly meals for students with allergies. This was a great relief! I soon after established a good core group of friends to go out with who understood my allergies and knew where I kept my auto-injector. Making the shift to university involves a lot of changes that relate to managing your food allergies. Taking smart measures can ensure both your safety and allow you to still make the most of your university experience!

*Quick Tip - Getting a single room can help you control what food comes into your room. If you want a roommate, though, requesting somebody you know is a good option. And, if you don't know your roommate ahead of time, it can still work well if you clearly explain your situation and how your roommate can help you.*

When things go wrong

**Learning Independence on the Fly, by Tess**
For the most part, going to university has been a great experience for me. But there have definitely been a few struggles along the way. The hardest of them has been moving away from home to another city. I now live four hours away from my parents who have always been there to help me when I need them. I didn't anticipate

how difficult things would be without that security blanket. It was an adjustment initially as I lived alone. But it was also a learning curve! I now have a great roommate who doesn't eat any of my allergens at home. She makes it easy for our little apartment to feel safe and just like home. I feel completely safe and don't have to worry about the contents of food or cross-contamination issues. At home, we never had my allergens in the cupboards. And that is the way that I like my new apartment cupboards as well. I couldn't imagine how it would be with a roommate who did want to eat my allergens. Likely it would be another learning curve. But I'm hoping that we will be together for the next few years and I won't have to adjust to that.

**Standing up for Yourself, by Sophia**

Even though we take as many precautions as we can, university is a place where we are completely independent and have to think and protect ourselves at whatever cost. College and university are really the best years of your life. And so they should be. However, having an allergy has made me realize how much more quickly I've had to mature, not only look out for myself, but also to stand up for myself. If you meet someone and explain to them how severe your allergy is, and they laugh about it and proceed to take out their peanut butter sandwich, there is not much you can do except walk away from the situation. I've learned that the most important thing is to stick by people who support you and your allergy and look out for you. Those people are your friends and you will want to have them with you if you are ever in a situation where you feel unsafe.

*Quick Tip - A college/university campus can be a huge place! Find out where the medical services are on campus and try to have friends around who know how to help in case of an emergency.*

## What would you say? (Q&A)

*Karen, Lindsay, Talia*

**How is the cafeteria situation at your college/university?**

**Karen** - There are so many cafeterias on campus. There are individual food service areas and individual seating areas. We have the options of sitting in large groups or in smaller groups at smaller tables. The clean up of dishes and garbage is left to the students. This poses the biggest risk. If a student eats something that I am allergic to, and leaves it on the table, I get uncomfortable sitting there. So I sometimes leave the area altogether and eat elsewhere.

**Lindsay** – Cafeterias are quite different in university than they are in high school. There are a wide variety of eateries. So you have plenty of options to choose from. At my school, all of the tables are kept quite clean by the staff. So I've never been concerned about cross-contamination issues. My school also does not have open peanut butter in any of the cafeterias. If you would like some, you have to ask for it and it comes in its own package. There are very few food items that actually contain nuts. This makes me feel very comfortable!

**Talia** - Personally, I always bring my food from home instead of buying it at the cafeteria. It takes a few extra minutes in the morning. But I know that what I'm eating is safe.

**What have you done to make sure you feel safe living in residence?**

**Karen** - I asked to get a single room so that I could control what foods were around. Because I did not have a kitchen, or any roommates, my room was perfectly safe for me. So I never had any problems. During the first day of the first year, we played an ice-breaker game. I always use this opportunity to highlight that I have food allergies so that people begin to become aware of it.

**Lindsay** - To ensure that I felt safe in residence, I notified my roommate well in advance about my allergies. I ensured that she both understood and was okay with living with somebody who had food allergies. When I first arrived at school, I spoke to my residence assistant who helped me make everyone aware at our first floor meeting. I was lucky to have two other people on my floor that also had allergies. So our floor mates were very understanding and respectful of our allergies. They were constantly on the lookout for any of our allergens that accidentally made their way onto our floor!

**Talia** - I live in an apartment, all by myself, and right near the school. I had previously lived with a roommate. But, after a few close calls, I realized that the risk of cross-contamination was just too high. I am more comfortable living by myself.

### Was your choice of school influenced by your allergies?

**Karen** - Yes and no. My school was influenced by my choice of program (which happens to be food-related). My allergies were a subsequent reason I chose my university. My school's hospitality services are great at catering to anybody's dietary restrictions, including allergies. You can literally pickup the phone, call hospitality services, and they'll make a meal specifically for you if need be. I was lucky enough that my school did not cook with my allergens except in pre-packaged baked goods. These are easy to stay away from.

**Lindsay** – My choice of school was not really influenced by my allergies. Choosing a school where I felt that I fit in and one that, obviously, had the program I wanted, were my main priorities. I did not want my allergies to have a major impact on such an important part of my education. With that said, when I went to tour all of my options of schools, I did make an effort to look into what it would be like with my food allergies and talked to the people in charge of food on campus.

**Talia** - I chose my school based on their great program. But I'm also lucky to be in a health-science program where everyone knows about allergies.

## How do you manage your allergies when living with friends/roommates?

**Karen** - I currently have two roommates who are great with the fact that I have allergies. My one roommate absolutely loves peanut butter. But, when we're away for school, she refrains from eating it at all because she knows that I'm allergic to it. I never asked her to do so. But she says it makes her feel better knowing that, by staying away from it, she's keeping me safe too.

**Lindsay** - I have now lived off campus for three years with roommates. I've never had an issue with my allergies. All of my roommates knew going into our house that they would not be able to have any of my allergens. They were all very understanding and totally okay with it. It is rare that we even have an item in our house that says "may contain." I am very fortunate to have such good roommates who really look out for me when it comes to my allergies.

**Talia** - My first roommate was a medical school student. So I was lucky that she understood how serious allergies could be. I mostly took the responsibility on myself to stay away from anything I was allergic to.

## Do you have any specific "rules" for roommates?

**Karen** – No. But I think I am just lucky that my two roommates are supportive and understanding. I introduced soy butter to my roommate who loves peanut butter. Although it's not the same, it's a great alternative that is similar enough to peanut butter. It is also safe to have in the house.

**Lindsay** – The only request I made of my roommates was to not have any items in the house that contain my allergens. They are free to eat them outside of the house. But I have asked them to ensure that they always wash their hands thoroughly before they come home. We have never run into any problems with this before.

**Talia** – My only rule for my roommate was to open a window if she was making fish. I'm allergic to fish and know that the aerosolized proteins can be problematic for me.

## Do you have many safe options with your meal plan?

**Karen** - The hospitality services at my school are super supportive of everybody's dietary restrictions and will work with you to find something that you can eat on campus.

**Lindsay** - I have a lot of safe options with my meal plan at school. My university does not serve any products containing nuts, except for a few baked goods. Hospitality services are extremely helpful for those with any dietary restrictions at my school. They post ingredient lists for any of their "homemade-type" meals and are more than willing to answer any questions you have. If you are having any issues, they will accommodate whatever your needs are.

**Talia** - I live off campus. So I'm responsible for my own meals. Of course, I only bring food into my apartment that I'm not allergic to. So I always feel safe.

## Did you find it really hard to adjust managing your allergies more independently without your parents?

**Karen** - I didn't find it too hard because my parents gave me more independence during high school to manage my allergies. I was able to just bring that with me to university. I have been lucky enough to meet a lot of people who understand the importance of anaphylaxis. But there are also people who are ignorant about it. But that's just life. I can tell you that I am more cautious because my parents are not around. Yet I am also more creative because university gives me the opportunity to try new things.

**Lindsay** - I didn't find it too difficult to adjust my allergy management when going to university. I think that a big part of having allergies as a child is that they kind of force you to become independent at a young age. While I was growing up, my parents really put an emphasis on me being able to manage my allergies on my own. They knew that, one day, I would be moving away from them. Therefore, I felt very prepared when I left for school. I haven't had any problems adjusting.

**Talia** - I think that, compared to high school, university has a lot more social events that involve eating (dinners, cocktail hours, etc.). Having to face all of those situations on my own has helped me learn how to effectively communicate my allergies to others. This was something my parents used to do for me when I was younger.

## To wrap it up...

The transition to college or university is a very exciting time! When figuring out how you'll manage your allergies, there are a lot of things to consider. But it does not need to be overwhelming because, with some preparation and research, the transition can be very manageable.

If you choose to live in residence, you'll need to figure out whether you want a single or shared room. Having a single room can make things easier; but, if you're living with roommates, it can work out really well as long as you tell them ahead of time and work together on some ground that everyone is on board with. Once you move into residence, you'll want to tell your floor supervisor about your allergies. And telling others living on your floor is also a good idea.

Getting a meal plan is often possible, even if you have many allergies, because meal plans have a lot of options and cafeteria staffs are usually pretty accommodating. They have to deal with many students with a wide variety of dietary needs. If you're visiting the school ahead of time, it's worth taking a trip to all of the eating establishments to see what they are like. Talk to the chefs or managers at each location to see what is safe for you to eat and if you can get separate meals made if necessary. If, after researching, you do not feel that a meal plan would suit you, there are other options such as choosing a residence with a kitchenette or living in an apartment on or off campus.

While in college or university, you may choose to live in a house or apartment with others, which can be a lot of fun and a great experience. When choosing your housemates, make sure they all understand your allergies before you choose to live together. You'll have to work together on finding ways to reduce the risk of being exposed to your allergens. You may wish to allocate cupboards so that you have your own space for your food or, alternatively, there can be one particular cupboard where your housemates can put things that contain or may contain your allergen(s). You can also offer alternatives to things you're allergic to, or establish designated cutlery, plates and pots that are only used for certain foods.

Overall, going to college or university is a time when you really experience independence. If you are moving away, you'll probably be meeting tons of new people. From the beginning, it is important to rebuild a network of people around you who know about your allergies and could help you if you had a reaction. Be confident that you know how to manage your allergies in different situations. Above all, have fun, study hard, and enjoy the experience!

## Summary Tips

1) Look into campus health and security and how they can help in an emergency.
2) Tell new friends about your allergies, including roommates and housemates.
3) Work with your campus cafeteria staff to find safe food options.

# Chapter 12
## *Dating*

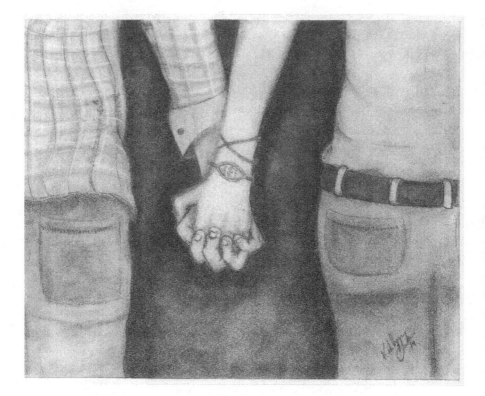

## Introduction

Dating is a normal, fun part of being a teen. But it can sometimes seem intimidating. As a teen with food allergies, it may seem even more daunting when you wonder things such as: "How do I bring up my allergies on a first date?" or "Can I kiss someone who has eaten my allergen if they brush their teeth?" or, as a final example, "Will my boyfriend or girlfriend have to give up my allergens completely?"

In any relationship, maintaining good communication is essential. Communication regarding your allergies is especially important since you both need to understand what has to be done to keep you safe. Generally, it is easiest to explain your allergies as soon as possible. At the beginning of the first date, or even beforehand, it is a good idea to explain what you are allergic to and what your date needs to know. Often it makes for a great conversation and it is usually much less awkward to tell them right away instead of waiting until the second date. If your date isn't willing to support you with your allergies, they're not worth your time.

## When things go right

### Surprise Allergy Aware Date, by Dylan

In my second year of university, I dated a girl who was great about my allergy. I had told her before our first date about the severity of my peanut and tree nut allergies and she followed up with questions about my auto-injector! She used to have a roommate who was a camp counsellor. So she was at least familiar with allergies through her roommate's stories. Anyway, on our first date, she wanted to go to a restaurant I had never even heard of. So I was quite hesitant to agree. But I didn't want to spoil her excitement. She sensed my hesitation and reassured me that she had already called the restaurant manager and spoke with the chef about my allergy. Everything on the menu was safe for me to eat and my date didn't even eat her usual peanut butter sandwich that day or the day before just in case one of us made the move for a kiss (which I did end- up doing). I couldn't believe how careful and thorough she was. All in all that was a great date experience!

### On the Same Page, by Tess

My boyfriend is really understanding and aware when it comes to my allergy. When he first met me and found out about my allergies, however, I think he was a little apprehensive and unsure of how to handle it. As time went by, he learned more and realized that it is easy to manage as long as the right questions are asked and the necessary precautions are taken. He makes a point of not eating anything I'm allergic to whenever we spend time together. On the odd occasion, when he has, he is always on the ball with telling me right away and washing his hands, etc. He is cautious about buying pre-packaged food when we are going to make food at his apartment and I think he actually checks the labels in more detail than I do! I feel that communication is a really important factor when it comes to dating with food allergies. It's all about figuring out a system between the two of you that works and makes you as safe as possible.

*Quick Tip* - *Having a new boyfriend or girlfriend read ingredients with you is a great way to make sure they fully get it. They'll probably have questions for you about specific ingredients and cross-contamination. But you can impress them with your expertise!*

## When things go wrong

**More than a Kiss, by Tess**

When I was dating my high school boyfriend, we definitely had more than a few mix-ups with my allergies. One evening, when we were watching a movie, he kissed me after eating one of my allergens in a snack that he prepared and ate in another room. After a few minutes, my face became extremely itchy and I ran to the bathroom to discover that I was covered in hives. As the symptoms progressed, I made the decision to use my auto-injector and was taken to the hospital. It was a really difficult and awkward conversation to have afterward, especially because we were both teenagers at the time. I had to stress how important it was to communicate what he ate when we were going to be together. At first it felt like asking too much but, when I thought about it, I came to the conclusion that, if he wants to kiss me, he's going to have to figure out what's more important—the snack or being able to kiss me. In my current relationship, we are older and I'm more comfortable about setting out the rules. It has become second nature. Good communication is vital when you are sharing your life with another person. And, when you add in a food allergy, it is of SUPREME IMPORTANCE!

## The "Allergy Talk", by Talia

Chris and I had been dating for a few weeks when I decided to have "the allergy talk" with him. I explained to him that I had to avoid certain foods and that even small traces of an allergen could result in a severe reaction. He told me I was overreacting and being a bit neurotic. Hearing him say that really hurt me, because it took a lot of courage to talk about my allergies with him. I really liked him, so I pushed the conversation to the back of my head and moved on.

A few months later, we went on a trip to Spain together. Needless to say, eating out with him was a challenge. He wanted to try crazy new foods. But, because of the language barrier and the scarcity of emergency medical services (we were visiting small beach towns), I stuck to basics. He couldn't understand why I wouldn't try new things and constantly pressured me to eat foods I wasn't comfortable with. One night, during dinner, he used his fork to try some of the spaghetti on my plate. I freaked out. I didn't know the ingredients in his meal and he had just contaminated mine. We broke up a few weeks later for different reasons.

What did I learn from all this? Most importantly, no matter how cute a guy is, if he doesn't take your allergies seriously, he is not the right guy for you. You deserve better. There are some amazing, caring guys out there who will understand your needs and be there for you no matter what. My current boyfriend understands perfectly and even carries my auto-injectors for me when my purse is full. I think the moral of the story is to not settle for a toad when your prince could be right around the corner.

*Quick Tip - When you become close with someone, you can really use it to your advantage with food allergies. They can be an extra set of eyes to read labels, a second opinion on an "iffy" dessert, and another helper to remind you to bring you auto-injector. Involve them early and often and it can actually make your life easier.*

## What would you say? (Q&A)
*Hannah, Lindsay, and Nick*

**How do you bring up your allergies when you are going on a first date?**

**Hannah** - It works really well if your first date is food-oriented. It gives you a natural pathway to discuss allergies. When you're looking at the menu, you can casually mention that you need to be careful with what you order because you have allergies, etc. But, if your first date isn't food-oriented, you have to just find a pause in conversation to stick the facts in. Keep it brief. But, if your date wants to know more, tell him or her enough without overwhelming them—or, worse, freaking them out!

**Lindsay** - I try to bring it up in a casual way when choosing which restaurant to go to or where to hang out. I try to make it not very intimidating or scary for the person I'm telling.

**Nick** - Personally, I think the best way to connect with another person is through getting a coffee together or going out on a dinner date. This works well for me since it is naturally a good transition point to mention my allergy in a regular conversation.

**Do you ever try to keep it to yourself that you have allergies?**

**Hannah** - Although it can be tempting to keep my allergies to myself for fear of spoiling the mood or drawing too much unnecessary attention, I never keep my allergies a secret. Allergies are a serious matter. But they don't have to stop you from doing things or ruin a perfectly good dinner at a restaurant. The key is to manage them with a plan ahead of time and that includes making sure the people you're with are aware of how they can help keep you safe.

**Lindsay** - I never try to keep it to myself that I have allergies. I might not bring it up until I know the person pretty well and begin to go on dates with them. Yet I never keep it a secret because that is very risky!

**Nick** - I don't think that would be a good idea. I wouldn't go crazy and talk about some tragic, emotional story connected with your allergy. But informing your date about your allergy can eliminate some bad situations in the future.

**Does your boyfriend or girlfriend stop eating your allergens entirely? Only on days they know they are seeing you? Other?**

**Hannah -** Different people have different ways of dealing with dating. Personally, I find it most comforting when my date agrees to stop eating my allergens entirely. That way I can trust that it will never be a problem between us. On the other hand, if your date isn't willing to do that, there's nothing wrong with allowing him or her to eat your allergen on days when you won't be seeing each other. This situation would make me a little nervous though just because I couldn't be entirely sure of how seriously my boyfriend was taking my allergies. Agreeing to drop the food entirely shows an understanding of the severity of the situation and eating habits can always be altered later once he better understands how allergies work.

**Lindsay** - My boyfriend is a vegetarian. So he cannot completely eliminate nuts from his diet as it's a great source of protein for him. He did stop eating peanuts since I am severely allergic to them. When he knows he is seeing me, he will try to avoid other nuts and will brush his teeth before we get together.

**Nick** - In the past, I wouldn't make my girlfriend stop eating my allergen entirely. I don't see it as fair on my part. However, on days we would do things or see each other, she would go out of her way to avoid my allergen.

**Have you ever had a reaction from kissing someone?**

**Hannah** - I have never had a reaction from kissing someone. But I know it is possible and can be a very serious thing. That's why it's important to tell your date about your allergies before things get very awkward very fast!

**Kyle** – I had a reaction after my girlfriend and I kissed. I had no clue where the reaction was coming from until I asked her what she ate that day. I found out that she had eggs (my allergen) for breakfast. Luckily it was not a major reaction!

**Lindsay** - I have luckily never had any serious reaction from kissing someone. There have been one or two times where I felt a bit funny. But it went away very quickly.

**Nick** - Nope. I can't say I have!

## Do you ask people if they have eaten your allergen before kissing?

**Hannah** - If you and your date haven't discussed your allergies previously, it is very important to ask what he or she has eaten before you kiss. If you want to avoid this awkward situation, just talk about it before the moment happens and that should smooth things over!

**Lindsay** - I try my best to do this every time before I kiss somebody that is not very familiar with my allergies or if it is somebody new I am dating. It can be awkward and embarrassing. But, if you are casual about it, and the other person likes you, it will be fine!

**Nick** - It depends on the situation of the kiss and how far the relationship is. If I have been hanging around them for a bit, I assume it is safe. But, if you are unsure, definitely ask.

## What would you do if your date didn't take your allergies seriously?

**Hannah** - If my date didn't take my allergies seriously, he would no longer be my date. Allergies are a part of me as much as anything else. And someone not taking them seriously shows a lack of respect for my health. I wouldn't be able to trust someone who didn't believe in helping to keep me safe. Not understanding allergies shows a lack of maturity. And not wanting to understand is just plain rude. If your date isn't taking your allergies seriously, you could be putting yourself in a risky situation. And you'll have to decide what feels safest to you.

**Lindsay** - I would explain to them how serious my allergies are and really emphasize how they are life-threatening. If they still didn't get it, or didn't take them seriously, I would stop seeing them.

**Nick** - For me, that is kind of a deal breaker. I would try to explain how serious they are. But, if they are still immature about it, the relationship would be over.

### Have you ever been too embarrassed to bring up your allergies with a new date?

**Hannah** - It's always a little embarrassing to bring up your allergies with a new date. But it's something that must be done. I've never been TOO embarrassed to bring up my allergies. I'm used to the little pangs of nervousness that come with the "allergy talk." If you want to be able to enjoy your night, it's best just to spit it out whenever the opportunity arises. Plus, the longer you wait to tell your date about your allergies, the harder it gets to bring it up. If you don't do it on the first date, it might feel even more awkward to do it on the second!

**Lindsay** - I have been embarrassed to bring up my allergies with a new date. To try and make it less awkward, I bring it up over text message and then talk about it again in person.

**Nick** - Personally, this hasn't been an issue for me. I feel that being as honest as possible with your date about who you are is a great thing anyway. If they reject you, because of your allergies, they aren't worth your time anyway!

## To wrap it up...

After reading this chapter, you've hopefully realized that dating with food allergies is very manageable as long as the right steps are taken to ensure your safety. The way you choose to handle your allergies with a date or boyfriend or girlfriend is up to you. But there are a number of important things to consider. You must realize that your allergies are a part of who you are and that your date needs to accept it. Never compromise your safety for a date. If they aren't willing to help you stay safe with your allergies, they are not worth your time. That being said, people will often be very good about learning how they can help you manage your allergies. So don't write them off without giving them a chance.

It is always a good idea to bring up your allergies early. There is no need to make your allergies sound scary. But it is important to state the facts, show your date your auto-injector, and make sure that they would know what to do in the case of a reaction.

There are a number of different ways of having a boyfriend or girlfriend manage your allergies with regards to whether or not they consume your allergen(s) and if there is anything they do before seeing you to ensure that you are safe. One way is for them to stop eating your allergens entirely. This is certainly a great way to make sure that you're totally safe and it works very well for some people.

It is great if your boyfriend or girlfriend agrees to totally avoid your allergen(s). Yet you may also decide that it is unnecessary as long as other precautions are taken. A good compromise may be for your boyfriend or girlfriend to avoid your allergen(s) on days you are seeing each other. If, however, they have consumed an allergen earlier in the day, you will have to be very careful before kissing. If it has been several hours, they have eaten other things in between, and they have brushed their teeth, it is probably safe. Some of this depends on how severe your allergy is as well, so having a discussion with a new boyfriend or girlfriend is important so you can figure out between the two of you what the best option will be.

Most importantly, be yourself! Whether or not you have allergies, people will like you for who you are. Your allergies are a part of you and need to be taken care of. But they should not stop you from having a great time dating.


## Summary Tips

1) Tell your partner about your allergies sooner rather than later.
2) Someone who doesn't take your allergies seriously isn't worth your time.
3) Be aware that kissing can be an issue if your date has recently eaten your allergen.

# Chapter 13

## *People Who Don't "Get It"*

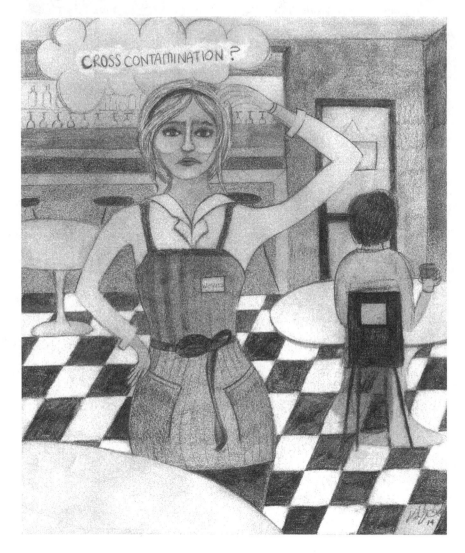

## Introduction

"Hello!? Is this the first time you have ever heard of food allergies?" Has that statement ever entered your mind when dealing with others? It's understandable that, if someone has never encountered someone with allergies, they might not initially "get it." In this day and age, however, doesn't everyone know someone with a food allergy?

It is really frustrating when some people think they know it all and downplay the seriousness of food allergies.

You know this frustration first hand if you have encountered people like this. It's like trying to explain math to a brick wall. Luckily there are some things you can do to help others understand and make this world a little more allergy aware in the process.

## When things go right

**Tea for Two...with a Substitute, by Erika**
It was the first day of our annual conference for National Millennium Scholarship recipients. The catering staff had tried to be understanding about my food allergies. However, they did not understand the severity of them. Nor did they have any ideas about how to accommodate them. Between the workshops and speakers, there were snack breaks where they served tea, coffee, and desserts.

At the first break, I decided I would ask if they had a substitute for milk (I was severely intolerant at the time). I am also severely allergic to soy. So I was hoping that they might have rice milk. I went to one of the servers, mentioned my allergy to soy and intolerance to milk, and asked if they had any other alternative besides milk. The server said they did. And, before I could ask him if it was rice milk, he had disappeared into the kitchen. When he returned, I asked him if it was rice milk. He said that it was soy milk. I had to explain to him, calmly, that soy milk would send me to the hospital in the same way soy protein or soybeans would. He said he was sorry and that he did not think soy milk would cause a reaction. I decided to take the opportunity to educate him about allergies in the hope that he would understand the next person who approached him about food allergies. Once I had explained to him what food allergies were, and how they could be life-threatening for many of us, he asked me if I would like him to get rice milk for the rest of the conference. I said 'yes', told him the brands I can have, and thanked him. He came up to me during the afternoon break with rice milk for my tea.

**Even My Butcher Gets It, by Katelyn**
I went through a particularly rough period of time trying to find a butcher that would accommodate my allergies to peanuts, tree nuts, peas, chickpeas and lentils. After trying multiple butchers in my area, who couldn't accommodate me because of cross-contamination issues, I finally found one! My butcher knows about allergies and takes every precaution to make sure that everything is to the exact specifications that I need. My butcher actually cleans the machines in the morning and packages (vacuum seals) a months' worth of meat for me. I am not the only person that he accommodates. He's had several people with allergies that he has helped upon request. My butcher is a really outstanding person and he has helped me out so much.

*Quick Tip* - *Keep in mind that you may actually be the first person with food allergies that someone has ever encountered. It's a great opportunity to help them understand what allergies are all about.*

## When things go wrong

**Bump, Set, Wait! By Bailey**
I have serious allergies to peanuts, nuts, and chickpeas. I also happen to play competitive volleyball. One time I was playing at a local tournament when my mother had noticed homemade peanut butter cookies being sold at the canteen. My mother politely explained to the woman working that I had serious allergies to peanut butter and politely asked her if they could please stop selling the cookies as I was worried about peanut butter getting spread around everywhere. The woman, however, said they could not stop selling the cookies because they were bringing in money

for the hosting volleyball club. My mother, who was slightly taken back by the woman's response, explained that my allergies were potentially life-threatening and asked her again if they could please stop selling the cookies. The woman once again refused and the cookies continued to be sold at the tournament. This woman clearly did not understand the extent of my allergies. Nor was she willing to make any compromise. This story highlights the importance of educating those around us about anaphylaxis.

**Speed Bumps, by Arianne**

Some people just don't understand the seriousness of food allergies. These people unfortunately come in all ages. When I was in grade school, I encountered countless parents and students who refused to show compassion or understanding towards my food allergies. Birthday parties always proved a stressful time for my parents and me. The fear of what will be brought to the classroom was always a point of worry. One specific parent refused to acknowledge my allergies. She believed that I was faking and was just a nuisance. On the day of her daughter's birthday, she brought in her favourite peanut butter cupcakes. Without realizing it, our teacher handed them out to all of the students. This incident forced me to be sent home for the day because they feared I would have a reaction. The parent refused to admit that bringing in a dangerous snack was a problem. Her lack of respect taught me the lesson that some people may never understand the seriousness of food allergies. This doesn't mean that you should ever stop educating and informing others about the severity of food allergies. There might just be a couple of speed bumps along the way.

*Quick Tip - Ask one of your friends who really "gets" your food allergies what makes them take your allergies seriously. This outsider perspective can help you when trying to explain your allergies to others.*

# What would you say? (Q&A)

*Katelyn, Mathew, and Sydney H.*

**What is the most ridiculous thing someone has ever asked you or said to you about your allergies? How did you respond?**

**Katelyn** - The most ridiculous thing someone has said about my allergies is that the warning statements saying the product "may contain" or contains is just something the companies "have" to say for legal reasons. They suggested that there is no chance of having an allergic reaction in these cases. They stated that, if I did end up having a reaction, I have my auto-injector and that I would be "fine" (on more than one occasion). My response to this situation is always the same. I simply tell them that this is not the case and that those warnings are there to keep me safe from reactions caused by cross-contamination. Consuming a product with a precautionary warning label is not worth the risk. And I simply don't feel comfortable eating it. In the end, no matter how they react to my response, I do what I feel is right based upon my experiences and education about the subject.

**Mathew** - When I was younger, someone offered me cheesecake with nuts on it. When my mom told them that I couldn't eat it, they offered to scrape the nuts off of the top of the cake. We politely explained that the allergy was severe enough that that precaution wouldn't be sufficient.

**Sydney H.** - When I was in grade eight, I actually had someone ask me if my allergies were contagious! I responded to them by explaining what allergies were and that they were most definitely not contagious.

**Why do you think some people can be so naïve about food allergies?**

**Katelyn** - I believe that some people can be very closed-minded about food allergies because of their lack of education about the subject. Most people I've met, who seem closed-minded on the subject, have never met someone or have never known someone with an allergy. Some think that they are similar to seasonal allergies and are not life-threatening.

**Mathew** – If you are not educated about the matter, you might not be open to learning. I don't expect these people to fully understand the issue. I take it upon myself to educate these people.

**Sydney H.** - I think the main reason for this is a lack of understanding. Although allergies are a rising health issue, a lot of people still don't understand the severity of them. I think people can also be closed-minded because they have never experienced it personally.

## How can you help someone "get it"?

**Katelyn** - Knowledge about food allergies is starting to gain momentum, especially in elementary schools. This is a refreshing change from when I was in elementary school. I believe that, the more that people know about allergic reactions, the more they will be receptive to them.

**Mathew** - I try to be as blunt as possible. I find that this gets people's attention and will prompt them to look out for their fellow human beings.

**Sydney H.** - When people do not understand my allergies, I usually just come out and say that, if I consume that food, it is life-threatening! I then explain the symptoms of anaphylaxis, how I feel when experiencing them, and the treatment that is required.

## To wrap it up...

There are, unfortunately, many people out there who, while they may have good intentions, just can't seem to grasp the severity of food allergies and how they need to be handled. Luckily, with increasing awareness in schools and in the community, more and more people do understand food allergies. But dealing with those who don't is still an issue and can be quite frustrating.

When someone doesn't seem to "get it," they often just haven't been given a proper explanation about what life-threatening food allergies actually are (and how serious they can be). When dealing with these people, it helps to be very straightforward with them and explain as clearly as possible what you are allergic to, what can happen if you consume your allergen, and what needs to be done to help you.

Sometimes, however, people still seem unwilling to budge. In these cases, often the person has another conflicting interest in mind. Try to see things from their perspective as best you can and see if there is anything you can do for them to make it easier for them to accommodate you. This sounds a little crazy, right? It's difficult, but it can be done. Compromising is often very effective. The person will realize that you are not trying to make their life difficult and that your allergies are serious enough that you are willing to go out of your way to help them so that they can accommodate you.

If all else fails, removing yourself from the situation may be necessary so that you stay safe. Often, however, by explaining yourself clearly and offering to help them, you will manage to get the person to realize the severity of your allergies and what needs to be done to keep you safe.

## Summary Tips

1) Try to turn the situation into a positive by educating them about allergies.
2) Keep in mind that allergies are very new to some people.
3) Sometimes a compromise is needed. But make sure it's not at the expense of your safety.

# Chapter 14
## *Bullying*

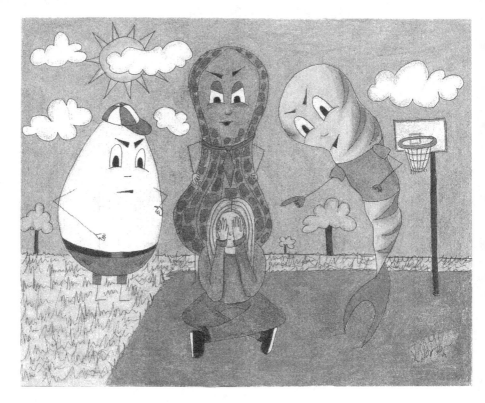

## Introduction

As you probably know, bullying can come in many forms and happen for many reasons. As an allergic kid or teen, you may have experienced bullying due to your food allergies (whether in the form of teasing or more serious harassment). It can be very difficult to stand up to bullying and to make it stop. But we hope that, in this chapter, you'll see that many other teens have experienced it and that you'll find some good advice about how to deal with it.

There are a few reasons why bullying due to food allergies may occur. Maybe the bully is channelling frustration about something they can't control. An example of this would be if someone blames your allergies and, ultimately you, as the reason why they can't bring peanut butter – or another food - to school.

Another reason is that the bully is simply looking for something about you to pick on. And allergies are an easy choice because they make you different. In minor cases, this may come as a comment like: "Oh, you can't have that... you're allergic. Too bad. It tastes REALLY good." This sort of bullying may come from their jealousy or their desire to put you down in order to boost themselves up.

The other main reason is that the bully may be curious or just not fully understand what allergies are. They may not know what it's like to deal with them or how serious they are. In this case, the bully may ask questions or make statements that seem stupid and sometimes a bit malicious, such as: "What would happen if I held a peanut near your face?" In this sort of situation, it is often helpful to explain to them how serious your allergies are and what can happen if you eat something you are allergic to. Don't be afraid to be firm with your explanations to make sure that they realize that your allergies are not a joke. In these situations, using humour can also go a long way as long as you make sure they are actually aware that your allergies are serious, and how ridiculous questions like these are.

## When things go right

**Graduation Party Invite, by Chelsea**
When I was in elementary school, my mom had always gone into my class before school started and made sure my teacher understood my allergy. I always carried my auto-injector on me and all of my friends knew about my allergy. In grade 6, a group of my peers were going to have a graduation party before we moved on to grade 7—which was in a high school. I had been close with these people throughout elementary school and I thought they were my friends. I found out that I was not invited to the party. It hurt my feelings and made me feel really bad because I didn't know why my lifelong friends wouldn't invite me to a party. One of the girls that was invited came up to me and told me I wasn't invited because of my allergy and because no one wanted to deal with it. I then felt even worse. I wasn't being invited because of something that I

couldn't control. I told my mom about it when I got home from school and she was very angry. Being chair of the parent committee, she talked to the parents about the girl having the party and told them about the situation. They felt bad because we all should be celebrating the event together. The next day, invitations went out to all the students in the grade. We then got to celebrate our graduation together.

*Quick Tip - Remember to express your feelings from the start. If you condone it when someone says something that makes you uncomfortable, what's to stop them from saying it again? Say how you feel or seek help in these situations.*

## When things go wrong

### That's Not My Name, by Jazmin

Even with all of the freely available information about allergies these days, some people still don't seem to understand allergies or take them seriously. I have been made to feel completely different from others in many situations because of my allergies. And, although there have been no big, specific situations that stick out in my head, there are many small things that really add up for me. For years, people called me "the allergic kid" instead of my name. That was difficult because my allergies don't define me. Are they a part of me? Yes. But I am so much more than "an allergic kid". People often say: "She's allergic to everything." This may not seem like a big deal. But, when they say it in a derogatory way, it feels like a punch in the face. In elementary school, I often ate alone. This in and of itself was a form of bullying. To a child who didn't understand why she was different, or why she had to be alone, it was difficult. One person once threatened to me with a joking tone: "What would happen if I snuck some milk into your lunch?" And, although I make many allergy jokes, this one crosses the line for me. I think most people with allergies have faced some sort of bullying, teasing or unwanted attention just for being "different."

Perhaps, when allergies are understood a bit more, the stigmas will slowly disappear.

**In a Peanut Butter Jam, by Nick**
During one summer, at a day camp, the local neighbourhood bully was sent there for the day with his lunch—a peanut butter sandwich. When lunchtime came, he was told he couldn't eat his sandwich due to the fact that I was there and I had a peanut allergy. In response, he decided to chase me with his sandwich to punish me for ruining his lunch. It was pretty scary running away from him! Luckily a camp counsellor spotted him and banned him from the day camp because of his actions.

**You Lack Discipline, by Arianne**
In grade three, I was coming to terms with my food allergies. Until then, I hadn't been allowed to eat lunch in the same room as the other children. Nor was I allowed around them during snack time before recess. But this year was different. I was finally able to sit and eat with my friends. However, other students seemed a little annoyed about not being able to eat what they wanted to.

One day, during lunch, a student brought a PB&J sandwich and, instead of me having to leave the room, they were escorted to another room to eat lunch. I guess they didn't appreciate the inconvenience because, over the next few days, she and her friends proceeded to taunt me and accuse me of faking my food allergies for attention. One day they brought it to the next level and hunted me down on the playground. Armed with a knife covered in peanut butter, they proceeded to hold me down and attempted to smear it on my face and mouth. Luckily a friend of mine saw these events and ran for a teacher.

The students were let off with a mere warning about the seriousness of food allergies and were sent home for the day. Our teacher made a small announcement about respecting food allergies.

After that, I became increasingly worried about my food allergies. I retreated back to eating alone and refrained from eating during snack time and going out for recess for quite a while. I became self-conscious and embarrassed about my allergies. It made me feel isolated and alone.

Looking back on the event, I feel that the school and the parents needed to reinforce the seriousness of food allergies to both students and parents to create a better understanding for everyone involved.

*Quick Tip* - *Your parents are always there for you if you are ever receiving unwanted attention or being bullied at school. Tell them early on what's happening and they can help you problem solve.*

## What would you say? (Q&A)
*Emily Rose, Giulia, and Sophia*

**Have you ever been bullied because of your allergies? What happened?**

**Emily Rose** - I was bullied mostly when I was younger. In grade five people used to toss wrappers at me of things I couldn't eat. As well, I would not be invited to birthday parties because of my allergy.

**Giulia** - When I was in elementary school, the students used to blame me because the school was nut-free. They thought it was my fault that they weren't allowed to bring peanuts or nut products into the school because of my allergy.

**Sophia** – I was bullied when I was in grade three and went to a new school. The kids would laugh and say: "Pumpkin seeds?! Yeah, right!" And I remember one girl bringing pumpkin seeds to class and shaking the bag in front of my face. Then she said she asked her mom to pack them for her because they're her favourite snack. Kids can be so mean!

**When did you experience the most severe bullying?**

**Emily Rose** - One time, in grade six, there was this boy who brought in something with peanuts in it for a holiday party. The teacher asked him to put it away. He didn't listen. He ended up making a big deal about it and getting called down to the principal's office. He yelled at me and said he didn't care if I died.

**Giulia** – It definitely was in elementary school. In elementary school, when you're a little different, the other students can really taunt you about it. It's also the age where people will do anything to fit in.

**Sophia** – It was probably from grade 3 up until grade 6. I think, when kids grow older, they care more about learning about their peers. And they realize what someone their age having a severe allergy really means.


**What sorts of peer pressure have you experienced regarding your allergies? What makes it so hard to deal with?**

**Emily Rose** - I have luckily never had negative peer pressure. All of my friends are very understanding and helpful when it comes to my allergy.

**Giulia** - Students used to say: "Oh, I bet you're not actually allergic to it. I bet you just don't like it and are ruining it for the rest of us." I wouldn't exactly call that peer pressure. But it affected my self-esteem negatively.

**Sophia** – The peer pressure I experienced regarded my "fanny pack." When you're younger, you don't carry around a purse or a bag everywhere you go. I remember my friends always told me to leave my pouch (with my EpiPen®) in my locker when we went to hang out outside. They didn't mean any harm; but they did not realize the possible severity of not having an accessible EpiPen® on hand.


**What are your favourite ways of standing up for yourself when someone says something unfriendly to you about your allergies?**

**Emily Rose** - I try to stay calm and explain how serious my allergy is to them. If they still don't listen, I try not to be around them as much or rely on them in an emergency.

**Giulia** - You need to act nonchalant and confident. If someone is unfriendly toward you because of your allergies, chances are that they just don't understand. It is your job to inform them about the severity of the situation and that it is not a joke.

**Sophia** – I try never to react in a negative way. When someone has something negative to say, I try to explain to him or her in a friendly tone what anaphylaxis really means. I use myself as an example and tell stories about my reactions in the past. It really changes their perspectives.

**Have you ever taken a risk that you later regretted because of peer pressure?**

**Emily Rose** – Thankfully not.

**Giulia** - Absolutely not. I was pretty good with not buying into peer pressure.

**Sophia** – Once or twice in grade school I left my EpiPen® in my locker and didn't bring it outside with me during recess. Even though my friends knew about my allergy, and knew where to find it, I realized after that it was a risk I should have never taken. I never did it again.

To wrap it up...

When bullying or teasing happens, we're often left wondering— why do people bully? It's one of those things about human nature that is very difficult to understand. Unfortunately, it does exist and we need to know how to respond to it so it doesn't get under our skin and affect us.

Although bullying may seem more common in elementary school, it can continue on into the teen years. You would think that people would know better by that age. Bullies can, however, be found in high schools, on sport teams, or even in the workplace. The important thing is to take notice when someone gives you unwanted attention. Use your voice and try to help them understand that what they're trying to achieve is hurtful and dangerous. Don't be afraid to get an adult involved if the situation escalates. Remember that allergies are not your fault and that you don't need to feel ashamed of them. Be confident about the fact that you have done nothing wrong and that you cannot, and should not, be the target of bullying.

## Summary Tips

1) Get help if you are ever teased or bullied.
2) Have confidence knowing that it's normal, common, and okay to have food allergies.
3) Stand up for others and don't be a bystander if you see someone being bullied.

# Chapter 15

*Educating Others*

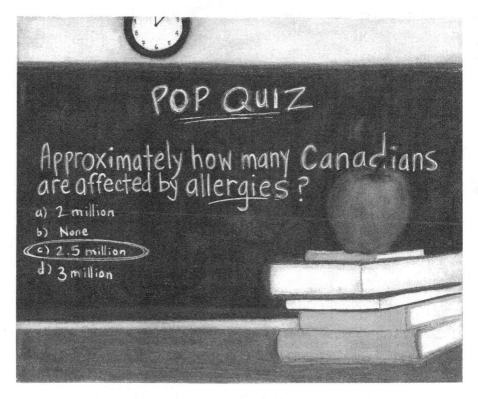

## Introduction

Building a network of people who understand your allergies, and who know how to help you, is one of the most beneficial things you can do as a teen with food allergies. As a child, your parents or other responsible adults are often there to help you out in tricky situations, warn you about potential allergens or ensure you are taken care of if you have a reaction. As a teen, you will find yourself more and more independent. But this does not mean you should have to deal with everything allergy-related on your own.

Educating others is incredibly useful. People who understand your allergies can help you out in a wide variety of situations. Whether you are having a severe reaction, having to deal with someone who doesn't "get it," or trying to figure out what restaurant to go to, it is always nice to have people to help you out and have your back.

Telling people about your allergies may sometimes seem daunting, especially if you just met them. It is always best to be honest and straightforward right away. Most people will listen and will be interested in learning how they can help. Educating people can be as simple as telling them what your allergies are. But it's often great to show them how to use your auto-injector, explain what a reaction looks like, and maybe even tell them about cross-contamination and reading ingredients. People are often fascinated to learn what you have to deal with and willing to learn more.

Finally, when you choose to educate friends, family, teachers, coaches or anyone else about allergies, you are helping to spread information that can change the lives of many people with allergies. The more people there are who understand allergies, the easier it gets for all of us!

## When things go right

**Two Steps Ahead of Me, by Bailey**

I always try to take every opportunity to educate others about anaphylaxis, particularly my friends. I try to teach all of my friends how to use my auto-injector and what to do if I was to have a reaction. But I've always wondered if they truly understand how serious my allergies are. One day, after school, a group of my friends and I were planning on going out for dinner. Originally, we were going to go to a restaurant where I had eaten many times before. So I felt certain that the food was safe for me to eat. At the last minute, however, two of my friends decided that they wanted to eat at a different restaurant that I had never been to before. When they proposed this idea, I told them that I would have to call the restaurant first to see if it would be safe for me to eat there. To my surprise, my friends then told me that they had already called the restaurant themselves and asked about all of my allergens. This showed me that my closest friends really do understand how severe anaphylaxis is and I hope that, in the future, more people will be able to understand it as well.

*Quick Tip* - *Building friendships with others who truly understand your allergies is really helpful in a variety of situations. You can build a great support system by informing others what your allergies are, how to read labels and how to handle a reaction.*

## When things go wrong

**Own Your Allergies, by Tess**

At the very beginning of grade 9, my French teacher brought in food to help expand our French experience. She did this without notifying our class or parents. As an afterthought, I think the teacher remembered that I had food allergies. So, at the start of the class, I was asked to come to the front of the class and to look at the samples of food that she had brought in. I felt a lot of pressure up there in front of everyone to decide about whether I could eat these samples or not. These items were from a deli, so the labelling was already rudimentary and absent on some items. I really wanted to fit in and feel normal for once. And I felt an enormous amount of pressure to make the decision quickly so that the class could begin. Ultimately, I decided that I could probably eat the food.

After eating some of the samples of food, I began to have a reaction. I notified the teacher immediately that I was having airway and throat symptoms. This was when the teacher made her second mistake. She sent me down to the office, alone, while a reaction was happening. In this situation, she completely ignored the school policy and my emergency plan. She provided food that was not approved, put me in the really awkward position of having to decide what was safe without all of the information required, and then she sent me down to the office in a huge school without any attempt to help treat the reaction or notify anyone that I was in need of medical attention.

There were several meetings involving the teacher, the school principal, and my parents following this situation. The events were examined to determine what mistakes were made and why my emergency plan and the school district policy were not followed. I think the teacher learned a great deal through this process and I hope she would act differently given the same sort of situation. What I want others to learn from this story is that you, as a young person, have to know what the steps of your emergency plan are and, if you feel you are having an allergic reaction, you need to "own your plan" and carry out the steps (whether or not the adults around you "get it" or not). That is to say, give yourself your epinephrine and direct someone to call an ambulance. Don't let others delay your emergency plan and treatment through their lack of knowledge. However, I realized the important lesson that I should not have eaten the food in the first place.

**Double Checking Everything, and Everyone, by Caiti**
I have always felt safe when it came to family members preparing food for me. Since I was diagnosed with severe allergies to milk, eggs, nuts, and peanuts at a young age, my family has always been very aware of the severity of my allergies. One thing that never occurred to me, however, was how family members may become forgetful as they age.

My grandparents have always baked for me for as long as I can remember. From cakes to cookies, they had built up a recipe book of allergy-safe baked goods. However, one afternoon, I was eating a Rice Krispy square my grandpa had made when my throat began to tingle. I immediately questioned what was in the square and my first thought was a possible cross-contamination situation. When I asked my grandpa to quickly review what he put in, he revealed that he might have used the wrong margarine. We went to the fridge and found that the margarine container he had used looked very similar to the margarine that is safe for me. The one used, however, was not safe. As the reaction got worse, I took my epinephrine and had him drive me straight to the hospital.

I knew my grandpa felt extremely bad about what he had done. However, I also took some responsibility for this. Knowing how the elderly can struggle with things like eyesight and remembering to read the ingredients, I should have been checking the ingredients as well. I guess growing up with my grandparents making me safe food for so long allowed me to let me guard down around them. From then on, I have started double-checking all ingredients when they cook for me.

*Quick Tip* - *Reminding people once in a while about what you are allergic to, how to use your auto-injector, and what to do in case of a reaction is very helpful—especially for relatives and friends you may not see very often. It's important to realize that, even though people have good intentions, it is easy to forget details sometimes.*

## What would you say? (Q&A)

*Erika, Katelyn, Sophia*

### How soon do you tell people?

**Erika** - I will tell new friends about my severe allergies right away. All my friends have known about my allergies from the very beginning of our friendships.

**Katelyn** - Whenever I meet someone new, I always make sure to tell them as soon as the opportunity presents itself—especially if there is food involved.

**Sophia** – I tell people when I am comfortable. But I tell them as soon as possible if there is food involved. There is no point in keeping it to yourself when you're in that kind of situation.

### Are your friends trained to use your auto-injector? How do you train them?

**Erika** - I have trained all my friends on how to use an auto-injector in case there is a situation when I cannot administer it myself. I have trained them using a demonstration auto-injector so they can practice administering it themselves. This helps them feel less frightened about possibly having to administer it on me one day.

**Katelyn** - I show any friend that I go out for lunch or dinner with. Or, if I go to a party, I make sure there is someone with me that knows how to use my auto-injector. I find anaphylaxis to be a good conversation starter and the other person usually finds the auto-injector pretty interesting.

**Sophia** - All of my friends know how to use my auto-injector. I remember teaching my brother as well when I was twelve and he was eight! We sliced an orange in half, shoved it into a cup face down, and used an expired EpiPen® to see what it really feels like to use. The most important thing I tell my friends is to **not** take the auto-injector out of the thigh right away. Instead, hold it in for several seconds.

**Do all of your friends know about your allergies? Which ones don't?**

**Erika** – All of my friends know about my allergies and the severity of them. Knowing that they know makes me feel safer.

**Katelyn** - Every friend that I have knows about my allergy and they will usually inform me if they have come into contact with one my allergens.

**Sophia** - All of my friends know about my allergy. If I don't tell someone about my allergy, it's likely that I don't trust them or I don't spend enough time with them to deem it necessary. And that's not really someone I'd call a friend.

**What are your favourite ways of bringing up the topic of allergies?**

**Erika** - I often discuss my allergies when I first introduce myself to a new friend. It is a part of what makes me who I am. And I'd much rather explain my allergies right away rather than have them find out when I am having a reaction.

**Katelyn** - My favourite way of bringing up the topic of my allergies is to simply just bring it up whenever the opportunity presents itself. It is especially interesting to talk about with fellow biology students at my university who can also contribute to the conversation about the complex anatomical and biological processes that are involved in an allergic reaction!

Sophia – For me, Halloween is the best time (I am allergic to pumpkin seeds!). However, if it is not October, I tend to ease into it by relating it to something else. If, for instance, my eyes are itchy, I will say "Well, hello again allergies! I have a severe allergy to such and such."

## Do your high school teachers and coaches know about your allergies?

Erika - My high school teachers and coaches were all aware of my allergies. On the first day of each school year, I always spoke to each of my teachers individually about my allergies and showed them how to use my epinephrine auto-injector using a demonstration epinephrine auto-injector.

Sophia - When I was in high school, the main office had a wall with a picture of every student with an anaphylactic allergy. Underneath each picture was their name, their grade, their class and, of course, their allergies!

## Have you ever had issues with family members who don't get it?

Erika - I've had family members who do not understand my allergies at all and others who have not fully understood the severity of cross-contamination or 'may contain' labels. With proper explanations, I have helped them understand over time.

Katelyn - Allergies are typically not an easy topic of conversation to bring up around people who think they know what is best for you. Especially when they have taken that role their whole lives— namely family! I wasn't fortunate enough to have relatives who really understood and cared about my allergies and, thus, I learned to take care of myself. This experience has helped me grow into the young adult that I am and given me the realization that, no matter how difficult any situation is, allergies or not, you can always learn something from it.

**Sophia** - There will always be people you meet who just won't get it (even though they really do care about you). My close family happens to be more worried about my allergy than I am sometimes. And I think that is great. If a family member does not take it as seriously as you think they should, tell them how you feel. If you feel unsafe eating at their house, pretending like you don't is not going to help you and they will never know that they are putting you in serious danger.

**What do you think is the best way to educate others about allergies?**

**Erika** - It is important to explain the severity of your allergies and give examples about what will happen if there is cross-contamination or if you eat something that contains your allergen.

**Katelyn** - The best way to educate people about allergies is to never stop trying and keep a positive attitude.

**Sophia** – Instead of making it out to be something scary, which might give people a sense that you're being paranoid, I usually try to keep calm and tell it like it is. When you keep it simple, and are knowledgeable, people want to listen and understand you.

To wrap it up...

As you may have gathered by reading this chapter, educating others around you about your allergies is pretty important. Telling people what you are allergic to is a good start especially for people with whom you spend a lot of time. It is also useful to explain details such as how to use your auto-injector, how to recognize symptoms of a reaction, and how to read labels.

Generally, it is easiest to explain your allergies soon after you meet people. Be casual about it, use humour, explain the facts, make sure that they understand that they are serious, and show them your auto-injector. People are generally quite interested to learn about what you're dealing with and how they can help. It's important to remember that these people may have limited experience and knowledge about food allergies. They may be more than willing to help out once they are given the right information.

## Summary Tips

1) When educating others, work with them, not against them.
2) The goal is to empower them, not scare them with information.
3) The more people who know about your allergies, the more support and help you'll have.

# Section C

# Attitudes & Emotions

# Chapter 16
*Proving You're Responsible*

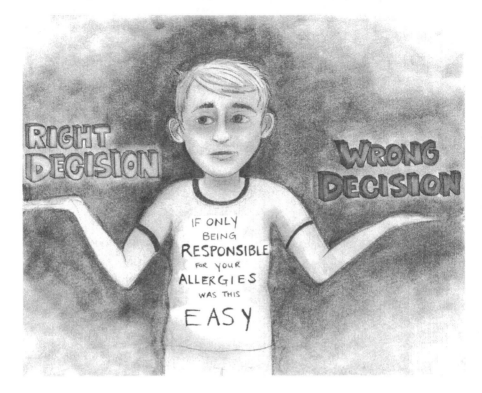

## Introduction

Within the past month, has your mom or dad asked you: "Do you have your EpiPen® or Allerject® with you?" If yes, this chapter is for you! Proving that we can be responsible enough to manage our own allergies is important. It isn't only important as far as getting our parents off of our backs. It is important to actually know how to navigate different situations by ourselves.

Keep in mind that taking care of your allergies has been a major part of your parents' lives. And they may have a hard time handing over the reins. Put yourself in their shoes. Think of your closest friend, or a pet, or a sibling. When asking someone to take care of them for you, wouldn't you want to be 100% sure that they know how? Proving to your parents that you can take care of yourself and your food allergies may take time, effort, and the occasional disagreement. However, we all want to be independent. And to do so usually means striking a good balance between demonstrating our abilities and having consideration for our parents' concerns.

## When things go right

**Handling Problems on My Own, by Chelsea**

Two years ago I started my first year of college and went to a school that was 2 hours away from home. This meant that I wouldn't be living with my parents anymore or have their protection when it came to my allergy. Living in residence, I had to get a meal plan and eat food from the caf instead of making my own food in my room. When going to the cafeteria, I realized that nothing was going to be peanut-free and that I would not be able to eat. This upset me a lot because I was hoping that something would go right while I was away from home. I also thought I had no choice but to pay for the meal plan (which meant I wasted $800). I went and talked to the person in charge of the cafeteria and she came up with multiple excuses about why they couldn't guarantee my safety. I knew I wouldn't be able to eat there ever and I wanted my money back. She told me to go talk to the person in charge of residence and see if it was possible. After making an appointment, I sat down with him and told him my problem and what I wanted. He understood the situation and told me a cheque would come in the mail for me with my full money back. I called my mom and told her what I had done. She was very proud of me and was glad I could handle things myself while being away from home.

*Quick Tip* - *Taking over the things that your parents normally do isn't easy. Remember that you can do things your own way as long as you don't compromise your safety. You can, for example, ask about ingredients in a different manner at restaurants and have your own way of showing others how to use your auto-injector.*

**Stay Focused, by Erika**

I was at a very allergy-friendly restaurant in Montreal, Quebec. It keeps its kitchen free of the top 8 most common food allergens. I was extremely excited to be going to this restaurant as I thought I would have an easy and safe experience. Still, I ran through my list of food allergies, and mentioned the severity of my allergies to ensure that they would take every possible precaution. I saw that they had bruschetta on gluten-free bread and got excited! I had not had bruschetta in years since going gluten-free. I ordered it as my appetizer and a steak for the main course. During this time, I was trying to maintain a conversation with my tablemates.

A few minutes later the waiter came back. He said that he had confirmed with the kitchen that everything would be safe and that they made the bread in house. As the waiter was placing the bruschetta in front of me, I had a flash. I quickly remembered that many gluten-free breads have pea flour in them (I am allergic to peas). I immediately asked him whether there was pea flour in the bread. He took the bruschetta back to the kitchen to find out. When I saw him walking back, he was shaking his head and informed me there actually was pea flour in it. Phew! Had I not clued in on the pea flour, I would have been administering my epinephrine and on my way to the hospital. It was a close call.

I was not focused enough when I was ordering because I felt this restaurant compared to other restaurants would be safer. And I thought that they would be more aware than other restaurants. I let down my guard and almost paid the price for it. Stay focused when speaking to the serving or kitchen staff. Distractions can cause mistakes. I learned in that moment that, every time I order, I need to be 100% focused and 'on my game'.

**Not all Carrot Cakes are Created Equal, by Nick**

Around the time that I was finishing elementary school, and moving on to high school, I started to assert my independence and started making decisions on my own. This included decisions surrounding my allergies to peanuts and tree nuts. One day my grade eight teacher was nice enough to bring some carrot cake. I figured that, because I ate my mother's carrot cake all the time, this cake would be safe. This was not quite the case. It was full of walnuts! After an injection, and a trip to the ER, I learned a great lesson: Always double-check and don't make assumptions.

**Revisiting an Old Snack, by Jazmin**

I have always been extremely responsible with my allergies and made sure to keep a close eye on ingredients. But, in grade 11, I decided to get a snack for my lunch that I hadn't had in a couple years. It was something that I always used to eat and was safe at the time. I was sitting in chemistry class eating my snack when, all of the sudden, my throat started to close off. I went to tell my teacher that I thought I was having an anaphylactic reaction and, as soon as I did, I lost consciousness. It was a very scary life or death situation and one that could have been avoided. I felt very embarrassed and responsible for the traumatic situation my class and my teachers had to endure. Although the ambulance came, and I was in the hospital for a while, one of my peers had read the ingredients of the snack I had been eating and, sure enough, there had been milk added to the ingredients list. That situation taught me to read every label even if I am used to eating it. Things change without warning and, lately, I have saved myself from many dangerous situations just by being tedious and extremely careful.

*Quick Tip* - *Reading ingredient lists on your own is a great way to prove that you're responsible. Better yet, call a manufacturer and inquire about the risks for cross-contamination for a product you are interested in. Simply explain that you are unsure about it.*

## What would you say? (Q&A)

*Chelsea, Emily Rose, Sydney H.*

**Do you ever feel that your parents are a little overprotective?**

**Chelsea** - Sometimes I feel like my parents are overprotective. As I got older, I realized that I am scared of more things than I should be. And I know that it is because my parents put very stringent guidelines in place for my allergy when I was younger—I have never stopped using these guidelines. I know now that it is hard being a parent of a child with allergies. You are continuously worrying about whether they are okay or not. It can come off as overprotective. But I realize that it's just because they want you to be safe.

**Emily Rose** - With my allergy, no. My parents have always wanted me to be independent and taught me how to be at a young age.

**Sydney H.** - Sometimes it can feel like my parents are overprotective. But that is just because they care. It can be annoying having your parents always asking if you have your auto-injector or if your friends know about your allergies. They, however, only want what's best. I am happy knowing that my parents care and are concerned for my safety.

**How have you convinced your parents that you are ready to take on more responsibility?**

**Chelsea** - I do this by eating before I go out, packing my own snacks, and calling restaurants ahead of time. I have also gone on trips without my parents and reported back the good things that have happened. And, if something wasn't perfect, I told them how I'd handled it. I've found that parents just want you to communicate and that they do not want you to leave them out of things.

**Emily Rose** - My parents can see how I handle my allergies in places such as a restaurant. So, when I go out alone, they trust me to do the same thing. They trust me enough to know I will not risk my life.

**Sydney H.** - I have gained trust from my parents by being a self-advocate. They know that I am responsible for my safety and that I can let teachers, friends, co-workers, and restaurant staff know about my allergies.

**How often do your parents ask you whether you are carrying your auto-injector?**

**Chelsea** - My parents used to ask me a lot when I was younger. But now they know I don't go anywhere without it. They trust that I have it. It is there for your safety. And not carrying it with you when you go somewhere could present a real problem if something does happen.

**Emily Rose** - Never... I start to freak out if I don't have it. So they don't bother anymore.

**Sydney H.** - Since my parents know I am getting older, and that I am responsible, they only ask every once in a while if I am going away for the weekend or to somewhere where there is a lot of food! Carrying my auto-injector has just become a part of my day-to-day routine!

**How do you feel when your parents second-guess how responsible you are for your allergies?**

**Chelsea** - I used to not be able to trust myself to ask the right questions when trying to advocate for myself—it caused a lot of anxiety. As I got older, my parents just learned to trust me and I learned to trust myself. It takes practice to know which questions to ask. And your parents are there to help you learn them.

**Emily Rose** - I'm lucky that this doesn't happen to me—that is a great feeling in itself.

**Sydney H.** - It can be frustrating when my parents don't trust me! But, by showing them that I respect that they care and are concerned, they realize that I am responsible and capable of taking care of my allergies.

**At what age do you think teens and young adults should be completely independent when managing their allergies?**

**Chelsea** - I feel that teens should be able to be fully responsible for their allergy when they go into high school. At this age, you start to go out with friends alone without parents and you're expected to be more independent about a lot of other things. It also prepares you for going away to school or moving out. You still have your parents if you need them in high school. But, when you go to university, they might not be as close as before.

**Emily Rose** - I think 16 or 17. This is because teenagers will be going off to university in two years. The two years gives them the safe space they need to learn and make mistakes.

**Sydney H.** - I think that all teens should be able to manage their own allergies since a lot of your teenage years are spent going out with your friends. It is, however, still very important to communicate with your parents about how you feel and if you need help with anything. They are there to help and this is great practice for when you go off to college or university.

To wrap it up...

Proving to your parents that you are responsible for managing your allergies yourself involves taking initiative and demonstrating to your parents that you are capable of managing different situations. Initially, it is important to demonstrate your ability to manage your allergies while your parents are around. For example, at a restaurant, ensure that you are the one who asks questions and speaks with the server, chef, or manager.

Starting off by showing you're responsible while your parents are present will allow them to feel more comfortable when you are dealing with situations on your own. When you do go out on your own, you may find it useful to be proactive and to explain to your parents exactly how you plan on handling your allergies wherever you are going. By doing this, they will realize that you have a good plan and they won't feel the need to nag or question you.

If you are going to a party, for example, you might show your parents that you have your auto-injector in your pocket and tell them about the two friends you are going with who also know how to use your auto-injector. If you are going out for lunch with friends, you could tell them what restaurant you are going to, who you are going with, what you are planning on eating, and where you are carrying your auto-injector. While this may seem over-the-top, it can be very helpful for the first few times you go out alone since your parents can see that you are thinking about different aspects of the situation and that you are taking the necessary precautions.

If you are still finding that you are not being given enough responsibility, you may choose to have a conversation with your parents explaining why you feel that you can be more independent. When having a conversation like this, it is important to be respectful and try to see their perspective. Explain why you are responsible and in what situations you would appreciate more freedom. And ask them how you can best show them that you know how to manage your allergies in these situations.

The process of proving that you are responsible comes in two parts: The first part involves learning the skills required to actually BE responsible. And the second part involves demonstrating that you have these necessary skills. It may take some time before your parents let you manage everything on your own. But, by understanding their point of view and explaining to them how you will take responsibility in different situations, they will be more and more willing to give you independence.

## Summary Tips

1) Want more independence from your parents? Prove that you can handle it!

2) Speaking about your allergies will show that you can advocate for yourself.

3) You will likely be asking about ingredients at restaurants for a long time. You might as well start early and get comfortable with it.

# Chapter 17
## *Frustration*

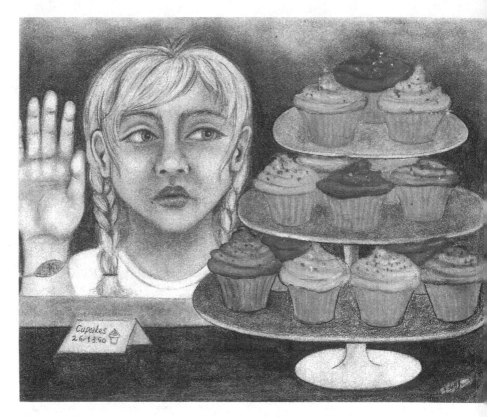

## Introduction

Someone has just offered you a delicious treat. So you ask to see the ingredients and read the label thoroughly like you do every time. So far, so good. Then, there it is - those few little words at the bottom saying "may contain [your allergen]." You know the feeling. We all do. And you're probably pretty used to it. But sometimes you still can't help thinking that it's unfair.

Maybe your friends want to check out an exotic new restaurant and you don't want to let them down. But you're pretty sure it'll be an allergen fest. Maybe your teacher brings in snacks for the entire class and they are full of your allergen. You feel both unsafe and left out. Maybe you really want to travel. But, in the country you want to visit, awareness about food allergies seems basically nonexistent and they speak a foreign language. Having allergies can certainly be frustrating in many situations.

Being frustrated due to your allergies is entirely normal and there are many teens with food allergies who can relate. Often, they find that they become less frustrated over time as they learn how to handle various situations and how to accept their allergies as a part of who they are.

It's important for you to recognize the things that make you upset or frustrated. And then you should backtrack and ask yourself whether these situations can be prevented altogether. Speaking to a party host in advance, having a translation card when travelling, having epinephrine with you or carrying a back-up snack may all be simple solutions to help you stay in control of an otherwise frustrating situation. And, you know that you can't change some people – like the ones who don't get your allergies – but you can change the way that you react to them, and choose not to get overly bothered by them.

## When things go right

**Window Shopping, by Stephanie**
The desserts looked spectacular. Beautiful morsels of sweetness and tasty treats of all shapes and colours—the kind that you only see in magazines—were spread out in front of me. I looked with awe... and then I took a step forward and looked closer. Most items had a sprinkling of the food that I am allergic to on them. If not, they were right beside another dessert that I was allergic to. This giant spread of desserts was pretty to look at, but I could not eat any of the desserts. I was "window shopping."

It can be very frustrating to have allergies and see everything in stores, bakeries, and restaurants that you cannot have. Instead, I try to appreciate what I *can* have. I do have a favourite dessert that I can buy at that store that is far away from all the things I am allergic to (and it is delicious). I have heard of allergen-free bakeries but, right now, I live too far away from any of them. One day I hope to venture to a city that has one—a road trip for cupcakes, perhaps?

I have also developed my baking skills and, although this takes time, I enjoy making my own treats and sharing them with others. I know that I will be able to eat at least one "safe food" at a party if I bring my own homemade dessert! Yes, it can be frustrating to frequently be "window shopping" when you have allergies. However, I use these opportunities to obtain ideas and inspiration for my next baking adventure!

**Healthy Eating, by Sophia**
Lately I've been trying to eat a lot healthier. I do not limit myself like many of my friends do when they go on "diets." But I do eat healthier things more often and unhealthy things in moderation. This has become difficult for me on occasion because I have a rare allergy to pumpkin seeds.

People tell me all the time: "Oh that's not as bad as peanuts!" That might be true in some cases. Peanuts and products derived from peanuts are used more frequently than pumpkin seeds are. Having a rare allergy, however, means that I seldom get a warning sign that I should not be eating something. Eating healthier is sometimes difficult for me because many producers are beginning to quietly incorporate pumpkin seeds into their foods. They have very powerful nutritional benefits.

Eating healthy means that I have to sacrifice eating certain granola bars, trail mixes and, most unfortunately, delicious breads. But, on a positive note, it also means that I can make them myself. If I see a delicious granola mixture with dried cranberries, chocolate chips, and pumpkin seeds, I can buy plain granola, dried cranberries, chocolate chips, and a pumpkin seed substitute, take those items home, and make something on my own that I know will be delicious and, most importantly, safe.

## When things go wrong

### Not a Sweet Experience, by Chelsea

During my grade 11 year, in high school, my dance class went to New York City for a week. We stayed at a hotel, went to shows, shopped, and went to dance classes. One day, after going to see a musical, we went to get a tour of the theatre and meet the actors. One of my friends really wanted to get a picture with the main actress and I told her that I would wait in line with her. After getting our picture taken, we realized that a lot of the class had left and we had to make it back to the hotel with a few of the other girls. On the walk to the hotel, some of the girls saw a huge candy store and wanted to go in. I told my friend I couldn't go in because of my allergy to peanuts (there was open peanut candy in the store). She told me she really wanted to go in and I would have to wait outside by myself. I told her it wasn't fair I had to stand outside alone since I waited with her in line to get her picture taken. One of the other girls started yelling at me and told me I was selfish for not letting my friend do what she wanted just because I couldn't. Not really knowing how to respond, I stood outside and waited for over 30 minutes. I felt so frustrated and angry at my allergy and the fact that I couldn't do everything everyone else did. It was a hard and irritating moment for me and, looking back on it now, I wish I'd stood up for myself instead of just taking it.

### The Bigger Picture, by Erika

In life, there will be things that do not go as planned. There will be times when we feel we are taking more steps backwards than we are forwards. I've had a significant amount of frustration in my life (most notably over the last few years). I've had to deal with injuries resulting from an accident on top of coping with my food allergies.

Food allergies are something that I have learned to manage. Speaking to restaurant staff has become almost second nature. I have done it so many times. The same can be said for reading labels. Even though I have experience managing my food allergies, having to deal with the chronic injuries from the accident on top of the day-to-day managing and coping with food allergies has given me more things to deal with.

I am not only living with life-threatening food allergies. I am also living with serious environmental allergies to dusts, moulds, and pets. I am also dealing with pain that does not go away. There are days where I am frustrated because it feels like I have so much on my shoulders. And I need to be careful at all times. I have to be "sharp" when reading labels, going over to someone's house for dinner or even having a friend over who has different food allergies. It is hard to have a clear mind when there is so much to "juggle." However, I have learned over the last few years how to be effective and stay on my game. When I am frustrated with all my health challenges, I remind myself that the feeling is only temporary and that I can deal with whatever comes my way. Having close friends and family you can talk to when you are frustrated is extremely important. They help you take a step back and look at the bigger picture. In moments when I am frustrated, my boyfriend gets me to relax and think about everything I have accomplished. He gets me to think about everything I have struggled with and overcome. And he reminds me that whatever I am frustrated with is yet another obstacle for me to overcome.

*Quick Tip* - *Different people have different ways of dealing with frustration. If you're feeling particularly frustrated, a few things you can try are writing it down, going for a jog, listening to music or talking it through with a friend. Figure out what works best for you.*

# What would you say? (Q&A)

*Bailey, Giulia, and Tess*

**Have you ever felt really frustrated because of your allergies?**

**Bailey** - There are times when I do feel very frustrated with my allergies. It can be frustrating when people don't take them seriously or when people get annoyed with me for not being able to go to a certain restaurant (as if it's my fault that I have allergies).

**Giulia** - Of course. Every time I can't eat something that everyone else is eating, or my friends go to a restaurant I know I can't eat at, I'm extremely frustrated. I am learning to deal with my frustrations as I get older. If my friends really want to go to a restaurant I can't go to, I let them go and I make other plans.

**Tess** - After so much experience with frustration and disappointment in the past, the only time I feel that I am frustrated is when I am attempting to explain my allergy to someone who just 'doesn't get it'. I try my best to turn those types of situations into learning opportunities. Overall, I feel like the people in my life are so accepting of my allergy that I often don't feel very different at all.

**What situations make you feel frustrated?**

**Bailey** - People not being able to comprehend the severity of my allergies frustrates me the most. I have been in situations where I have explained my allergies to someone and then they have eaten my allergen when I'm with them. This is extremely frustrating and also triggers my anxiety.

**Giulia** - I feel most frustrated when everyone else around me is eating something and I know I can't eat it—especially when someone says how good it is.

**Tess** - I get frustrated when people don't comprehend how serious my allergies are. In the long run, I find that those who have limited knowledge in the allergy area, and who aren't interested in learning, don't make long-lasting friends. The people I choose to surround myself with do get it and make my life easier, not more frustrating.

**What do you do to feel better and let off steam?**

**Bailey –** I always find I feel better after I work out and play sports. It's always been a good way for me to get my mind off of things.

**Giulia -** I try not to surround my social life with food. Go to the movie theatre, go dancing, and shop! You can have a lot more fun doing other activities.

**Tess -** I love to do any kind physical activity if I need to blow off some steam. If I'm still upset after that, I always find talking to someone about my frustrations helps. Whether it is my parents or a friend, I always find that they have useful words of wisdom.

**Is there anything you do to prevent feeling frustrated because of allergies?**

**Bailey -** I try to avoid situations where I would normally feel frustrated. You often have an idea of what has been frustrating in the past. So I use my experience to try and avoid that situation again in the future.

**Giulia -** You've got to let it go. You can't let it bother you too much. Be happy with what you have and the things you can do. Try not to let the things you can't do constantly cloud your mind and judgment.

**Tess -** In general, I think that knowing who to surround yourself with is a key aspect of a having a happy and healthy life. This is even more important when you have allergies. Being able to look at the big picture is a huge asset to have in your back pocket. It's not worth getting upset over the little things.

## To wrap it up...

Being frustrated with your allergies is completely normal. And it can happen in a variety of situations. It can be frustrating to see other people eating everything every day while we have to avoid so much because we developed food allergies - something we have no control over. It is okay to feel frustrated. But it is important to recognize what causes you to feel frustrated so that you can better cope with these feelings. You may find yourself frustrated because of a particular incident or situation. Or maybe you are just frustrated with the fact that you have allergies in general. If you know you're heading for a situation that may be tough to handle, prepare ahead of time as best you can. If you're simply feeling frustrated with having allergies, that's okay. However, taking a step back to think about everything that you are thankful for can help put things in perspective. Take a look at the chapter about "Seeing the Bright Side" for more helpful tips that may help with frustration.

## Summary Tips

1) It's normal to feel frustration when feeling emotional about your food allergies.
2) Find activities that help you deal with frustration.
3) Plan ahead for events that could cause possible frustration by bringing your own food.

# Chapter 18
*Anxiety*

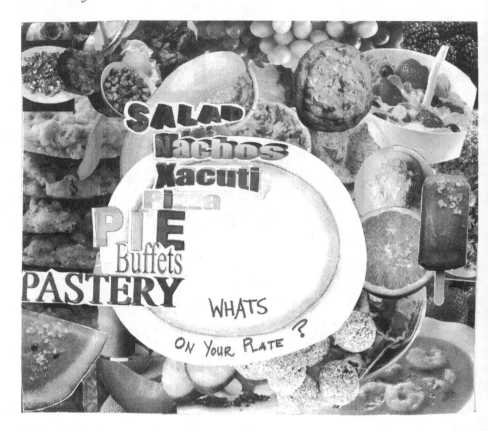

## Introduction

Feeling anxious about managing food allergies in different situations is common. We all know how serious allergic reactions can be and want to do everything to avoid them such as making sure what we eat is safe.

The good news is that food allergies are manageable and people can live happy, productive, and fulfilling lives. While it's important to recognize our fears and worries, it is equally important to keep risk in perspective, address them directly and understand how large the risk really is. Digging into current food allergy research is a great way to discover the true facts about food allergies and give confirmation on areas you were unsure about. You may be surprised to find that some of the information you may have received to be out of context or viewed as a myth compared to a reality.

There sometimes seems to be a fine line between taking risks and staying safe. It's key to learn how to tightrope walk along that line. Recognizing risks on one side and precautions on the other is necessary to help us balance our minds and emotions. Reminding yourself that you will be okay if you avoid your allergens and carry your auto-injectors is a good way to keep anxiety in check.

## When things go right

**Conquering Anxiety, by Sebastian**
Throughout my whole life, I have always been a very nervous person and been affected by anxiety on some level. Whether it was talking in front of my class, doing an assignment, or dealing with my allergy to peanuts, tree nuts, and penicillin, it hasn't always been easy. But that doesn't mean that I haven't overcome the problems I've faced. The anxiety that I have with allergies was especially strong when I was younger (around age 10 and 11) and when I felt most exposed to my allergens. This would mostly happen when I was at a restaurant. I would always check whether the food was safe or not. But I would always think that they were wrong and that they had no control over their food. The truth was that they had the most control of anyone. I would get so worried that I couldn't stay in the building and felt as though I had to get out of there. It was with the reassurance of my family that I was able to put everything into perspective and get my anxiety under control. Now, I hardly ever worry about my allergies. All I had to do was realize that I was doing the right things to stay safe and realize that the people around me didn't want me to have an allergic reaction.

### Ingredient Check Before Kitchen Prep, by Samantha

Luckily, I've had mostly good experiences at restaurants. I have had a couple of bad experiences. But I usually enjoy my time at restaurants because I am always really careful. I went to a new restaurant one time. It was a different type of restaurant than I normally go to. So I was nervous. We called ahead to make sure they could accommodate me and we looked at the menu online. When we got to the restaurant, the first thing I did was tell the waiter about my allergies. He immediately went to get the manager. When the manager came, she told me, in general, what I could eat and what I couldn't. After I ordered my meal, they went to the back and checked every ingredient to make sure it was safe. They also cooked my meal on a separate grill that hadn't been used since it had been washed the day before. Overall, I had a great experience and they were great with my allergies.

*Quick Tip* - Anxiety usually stems from uncertainty. So ask a lot of questions when you are unsure and you will hopefully feel better with more knowledge about the situation.

## When things go wrong

### May Contain Anxiety, by Sebastian

When I was in Grade 7, our class was going on a field trip to a camp for the week. When I found this out, I was extremely nervous seeing as I hadn't gone to many overnight camps. The idea of leaving home worried me. But the idea of having an allergic reaction terrified me. My parents always said: "You're going to be fine. You've never had an allergic reaction and it is very unlikely that you will." I naturally believed them (like I do to this day). My parents then checked to see if it was peanut and nut free and, luckily, it was. I decided to go on the trip and, for the most part, it was fine. The food was good, the activities were fun, and I was surrounded by wonderful people who looked out for me.

But, one day during lunch, I was eating a piece of bread and one of the counsellors came up to me and said: "Hey, Sebastian, did you check the bread before you ate it because we read the label and it said it "may contain peanuts?" I instantly froze. A thousand thoughts poured through my mind and I completely broke down. Luckily, I didn't have a reaction. But the anxiety was getting to my head. I kept thinking, "Is this the reaction or a panic attack?" I had never been in this situation before. I was fine in the end. But the most important thing to take out of this story isn't to be afraid of every situation you face. The most important thing to take from this story is to just be careful because there will always be situations like this. If, however, you stay calm and keep your head cool, you'll be in a better position to deal with it the next time.

**Fingers Crossed about the Restaurant, by Mathew**
The feeling of anxiety in regards to my allergies doesn't always relate to the potential consequences of coming into contact with an allergen. My anxiety is often triggered by having to deal with a situation publicly. Although I have many years of experience in terms of dealing with my allergies, I will sometimes become nervous when I have to make the decision to sit out of certain activities or make an inquiry to keep myself safe. Recently I was invited to an important dinner meeting. The person organizing the dinner was deciding where to hold the meeting. I instantly felt some anxiety because I knew that I might have to tell them that where we go may depend upon my allergies. I decided to not say anything and deal with the potential issue at the restaurant. I am lucky that we went to a restaurant that I knew to be very accommodating. Anxiety is a very difficult emotion to deal with. I recommend being conscious of it because, if you are aware of your anxiety before and when it is kicking in, you will have a better chance of overcoming it. Typically, if you have a significant amount of experience dealing with allergies, you will know what decisions to make in certain situations. Because of this, you will be less likely to make an emotionally-driven decision, even when anxiety kicks in.

## What would you say? (Q&A)

*Chelsea, Mathew and Stephanie*

**In what situations are you the most anxious when dealing with your allergies?**

**Chelsea** - Situations that make me the most anxious about my allergy include when I have to go to other people's houses for dinner. I feel like I can never trust anyone with my allergy and that cross-contamination can always be a problem. I usually eat before I go anywhere just to make sure. And, if I know the people, I decide whether I am eating beforehand using how much I know about how the food will be prepared to judge how safe it is. Although it makes me feel bad and rude for not eating, I have to do what I have to do to not have an anxiety attack.

**Mathew** - I feel most anxious when I am in a situation that could be dangerous or when there may be negative consequences if I speak up. Some people, for example, do not understand what an allergy is and I tend to be very anxious when they offer me food that is dangerous. I fear that, if I have to turn it down, they may think that that I am lying to avoid their offering of food.

**Stephanie** - I am most anxious in new restaurants that I have not tried before or at conferences or meetings where I cannot order food in advance. I just have to hope that they can accommodate my allergies.

**Who are the people you count on to be supportive?**

**Chelsea** - The people I depend on to be supportive are my parents and friends. They all know about my allergy and I expect that they won't put me in dangerous situations. And they understand when I say that I can't eat at places because of it. I also expect my boyfriend to be supportive. I spend most of my time with him and, if he didn't understand, it would be hard for me to feel safe around him.

**Mathew** - I count on my family and my friends who understand my allergies. Although you cannot rely on anyone but yourself, the support of the people who are close to you will give you the needed confidence to deal with your allergies effectively. If I have to speak up in a restaurant, I find it much easier to do around friends who understand my allergies than people that I have met for the first time.

**Stephanie** - I count on my friends and family to be supportive. A strong support network will help in the toughest situations (and they should always know where to find your auto-injector).

**Are there specific triggers that bring on anxiety for you?**

**Chelsea** - Some triggers that bring on anxiety are when people talk about my allergy when I am eating or when people around me have nuts. I also get anxious when I go to restaurants and the server doesn't seem 100% positive about my food being peanut-free. I usually leave or ask to speak to the manager because being safe is my number one priority.

**Mathew** - The worst trigger is seeing or smelling nuts while I am eating. My body must think that they are going to be ingested.

**Stephanie** - If I hear, "You could have an allergic reaction from this," then I get anxious. Sometimes that can happen at the doctor's office with a new medication or when getting a routine immunization.

**Have you ever had a panic or anxiety attack? How does it feel?**

**Chelsea** - I have never had a panic attack about my allergy. But I have stopped eating for days because of it. Feeling so unsafe that you refuse to eat does not feel very good. My parents have talked me through it multiple times and it has gotten to the point where I have made myself sick. The best advice I can give is to think logically about why you're not eating.

**Mathew** - I don't think I've had a full-on panic attack. But I have felt overwhelmed by anxiety. In those situations, I find that I have to bite the bullet and act on the anxiety. I know the anxiety is my body telling me that there is something wrong.

**What do you do to feel better?**

**Chelsea** - To get over my anxiety I usually have to talk to my mom or someone I know that will talk me through it. They usually tell me to think logically, to ask questions, and to remember that my allergen is not going to jump off the plate at me. If I can't talk to someone, I breathe deeply and tell myself to remain calm.

**Mathew** - I feel better by tackling my anxiety through "self talk" and reminding myself that the risks are minimal. This helps me conjure the confidence I need to stay level headed about the situation I am in.

**Stephanie** - I try to focus on something else and distract myself if I feel anxious. I think about other things I have to do, plans for the weekend or I just call a friend.

**What advice would you give to someone with anxiety about their food allergies?**

**Chelsea** – Think ahead. If you know you are going out to a restaurant where menu options might cause you problems, call ahead and ask about foods with your allergens. Alternatively, you can speak to a server before you sit down at the restaurant to make sure. Bring snacks wherever you go so you will always have something on you when there are not 100% allergen-free snacks around. And, of course, always carry your auto-injector!

**Mathew** – Preparation and research are the keys to tackling anxiety. They help by making you informed ahead of time. You could, for example, read the menu online ahead of time. You may find out that nothing but the desserts have your allergens and that the desserts are shipped in by a third party. This doesn't guarantee your safety. But at least you'll have more information to base your questions on.

**Stephanie** - Having food allergies can certainly cause you to be anxious (and for good reasons). I am often afraid to try new foods because I am scared that I will have a reaction to them. I recommend having a strong support network and getting involved in many different things so that you are not just focused on your allergies. Try to be prepared with your auto-injector and ensure that those around you know how to use it. An allergic reaction can happen at any time. But you do not have to let the fear of having one limit you from doing some amazing and spectacular things!

To wrap it up...

The situations that cause anxiety are often the ones where we feel unsure about our surroundings. We might feel a lack of familiarity and comfort or a lack of control over the situation in general. This can occur, for instance, if we don't know who is preparing food and whether they are aware of food allergies.

Remember that you can reduce your anxiety by taking precautions. Remind yourself that you'll always be okay as long as you take steps to reduce the risks asking about food preparation (and reading labels), by always carrying your auto-injector and knowing what to do in case of an allergic reaction. We all know, however, that there are situations that we just can't control. These tricky situations can happen. And this is when you have to be extra careful with your allergies. These situations are only temporary and can be prevented through precautionary measures like bringing your own food or avoiding eating altogether. You may wish to speak to a counsellor or a therapist if your anxiety is really becoming a persistent problem.

## Summary Tips

1) It's normal to feel anxious. However, keep reminding yourself that food allergies are manageable.
2) Have doubts and questions about situations or restaurants? Research more info or connect with others who may be able to help you get more information to learn the real risks involved.
3) Take things slowly and stay within your comfort zone as you try different restaurants and get into new situations.

# Chapter 19
## *Recovering Emotionally After an Allergic Reaction*

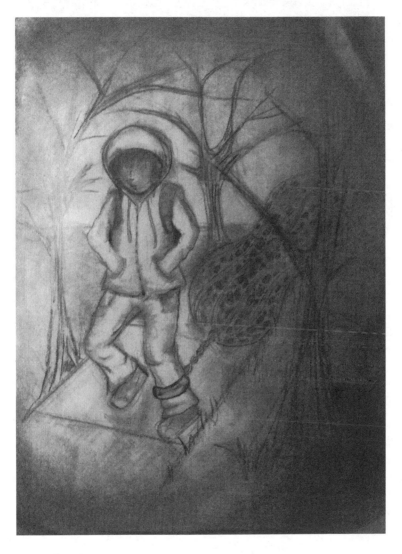

## Introduction

If you have never experienced a severe allergic reaction before, count yourself lucky. We all know that accidents can happen and that situations can sometimes be out of our control. Having an allergic reaction is nothing to be ashamed of and, although many reactions are preventable, often unexpected and unusual circumstances contribute to the situation. Beyond the physical symptoms, an allergic reaction can bring on a range of emotions both during and after the fact.

It can be pretty overwhelming to go from a normal meal to using an auto-injector, riding in an ambulance, and visiting the emergency room. Following the reaction, it is normal to feel uneasy, anxious or generally a little "off" after everything you've been through. The recovery process may take a little while and that is okay. There is no right or wrong way to recover emotionally after a reaction. Just remember that it's normal to feel shaken up. But you will be okay. Many others have been through and overcome similar emotions after experiencing a serious incident like a life-threatening reaction.

## When things go right

**An Ironic Reaction, by Erika**
I was on my way to an allergy and asthma conference. I had time before my flight and decided that I would grab a salad at the restaurant before going through security. I wrote down a long list of my food allergies and explained cross-contamination to the server. Unfortunately, even though she had assured me that everything would be fine, I suffered an anaphylactic reaction. I administered the epinephrine auto-injector and the restaurant called 9-1-1. They monitored my vitals once I was at the hospital. The conference was starting the next day and I did not want to miss it. I had experienced so many emotions, notably anger, fear, and sadness that I missed my flight and would spend the night in the hospital.

Spending a few hours at the hospital on my own gave me time to reflect. I thought about the fact that I had taken all the necessary precautions and that it was beyond my control. I concluded that I would never eat at an airport before a flight again. I reasoned with myself that it was not worth the risk and considered it a learning experience. I tried to relax. Everything was okay. I was at the hospital, doctors were taking care of me, and I would be on the next flight out to Quebec City. I did not have much time to dwell on what had happened. I needed to focus on getting myself on the plane. When the doctors gave me the green light to leave, my friend picked me up and we drove to the only pharmacy in town that was open. We filled my prescription for a new epinephrine auto-injector as I needed to have a second one with me. I told myself it was a "bump in the road" or "minor detour." I was not going to miss the conference nor was I going to miss seeing my family. I put the events behind me and boarded the plane with a clear head.

My family took me to the hotel once I arrived in Quebec City. We laughed at the irony that I had an anaphylactic reaction on the way to an allergy and asthma conference! My story was the talk of the conference. I learned that the best thing to do after a reaction is to reflect and then move on. It is important not to be stuck in a negative headspace. Staying positive is always the best course of action.


**Recovering Physically and Emotionally, by Karen**
I once had to leave work early because I was not feeling well. I did not realize that I was having an allergic reaction because the symptoms were not what I recognized. So, when I had to stop in the middle of the sidewalk to give myself epinephrine and call an ambulance, I felt so overwhelmed by everything. Having a reaction can take a toll on someone, especially when they least expect it and when they are alone. Sometimes having a reaction can make you feel like a failure because you always manage to stay safe — except for that one time you have a reaction. If I ever have a reaction, I always take the time afterwards to reassure myself that I am okay. I tell myself that I have taken the right steps and that I did the right thing. After this particular reaction, my parents drove me home and I just relaxed for a bit and recovered physically. Emotionally, I found it helpful to walk through the day in my mind to see where things went wrong. I know that it can be difficult. But I find it to be a learning process for the next time the situation might arise. I know I'll be prepared for it if it happens again.

## When things go wrong

### Not an Easy Recovery, by Bailey

Recovering from anaphylactic shock is different for everyone. But I think many would agree that the emotional recovery is far more difficult than recovering physically. When I was thirteen, I had an anaphylactic reaction to a cookie that contained one of my allergens. I did not recover well emotionally. After my reaction, I was paranoid that I was going to have another reaction and would have an anxiety attack every time I ate, even if the food was homemade. There were days when I just didn't eat at all to save myself the exhaustion that came along with these anxiety attacks. In time, I got more confident with my allergies and curbed the anxiety. But it took a while for me.

### What would you say? (Q&A)
*Daniela, Erika, Karen and Sydney H.*

### Does an allergic reaction take a toll on you emotionally?

**Daniela** - After my first severe reaction, at age ten, I found that it took a bit of a toll. I was a little more nervous eating away from home for a week or so. My second severe reaction at age sixteen, however, actually boosted my confidence a bit since I realized that using the auto-injector really isn't that hard and, by the next day, I felt back to normal.

**Erika** - After an allergic reaction, I often go over the details leading up to the reaction and try to figure out what I could have done differently to avoid the reaction. This does take a toll on me emotionally because I tend to blame myself or feel upset. However, I realize that there are times when even the most stringent precautions may not prevent a reaction from occurring.

**Karen** - Yes, it normally takes a day or two for me to get back into my normal habits. I become very cautious and aware of what I am eating and what utensils I'm using because of the thought of having another reaction.

**Sydney H.** - Most definitely! Anaphylaxis can be very frightening and can be very hard on you emotionally. After a reaction, I am usually pretty worked up and don't want to be alone. It can be hard to understand what you just went through and how it all happened so quickly.


**What do you do to recover and start healing/feeling better?**

**Daniela** - I like to move on quickly and continue with my normal routine so I do not dwell on the incident. I make sure to take time, though, to acknowledge what happened and learn from the experience.

**Erika** - After a reaction, I take some down time away from work, school, and other activities. I take some time to rest and let my mind and body recuperate because an allergic reaction takes a toll on my body mentally and physically.

**Karen** - I go home and usually keep to myself. I do not like when things go wrong. So recovering from an allergic reaction sometimes feels like I have failed myself. In reality, I know that I just took a misstep, which can happen on occasion. To start healing, I accept the fact that I am okay and I tell myself that I just need to be more cautious. Once I realize where everything went wrong, I figure out a way that I could have prevented it for the next time the situation may pop up.

**Sydney H.** - To emotionally recover after a reaction, I find it is best to get a lot of rest and never rush back into working or going to school. Give yourself time to process what you have been through to physically and emotionally heal. Also, talking about your feelings is very important. Whether it's a parent, sibling, or friend, talk about how you emotionally felt during the reaction and any fears that you now have. Getting stuff off of your chest is very important.

## How long does it take to get back to normal?

**Erika** - It can take a few weeks to get back to my usual self after a severe allergic reaction because I feel tired and weak.

**Karen** - It can take a few days for me to get back to normal, especially back to my normal eating habits. I become super conscientious about what I am eating immediately after a reaction, even in my own home where I know everything is safe. But this amount of time can differ for everyone. So it is hard to justify a set number of days for someone to get back to normal after having an allergic reaction.

**Sydney H.** - It all depends upon the severity of the reaction and the medicines you are prescribed. The day after, epinephrine can give you what I like to call "an epinephrine hangover" and leave you feeling pretty drowsy and wiped out. Stay positive, rest, and you will be back on your feet in no time.

## What advice would you give to someone who just had a reaction?

**Erika** - I would tell them to take some time to relax and to try not to blame themselves for what happened. Instead, they should focus on what they did right and what they could have done differently. I would tell them that they did well in terms of acting fast with the epinephrine auto-injector and seeking emergency medical treatment. I would also say that they need to focus on the positives.

**Karen** - I would tell them to walk through the day (if it's not too difficult for them). That way they can pinpoint what happened and find a way to prevent it next time. Emotionally, I would tell them to relax and try to get back into their normal habits as soon as they can. It's easy to dwell on something that can be as overwhelming as having an allergic reaction. But it's easier when things are back to normal because that's just what you do on a day-to-day basis.

**Sydney H.** - I would tell someone who just had a reaction that they are not alone and that there are a lot of people like them who have gone through the same thing. It is very scary. But remain positive and thankful that you are okay. It is also important to avoid dwelling on what you could have done differently to prevent the reaction; be thankful that you're okay! And, of course, remember to let your body rest after a reaction! You have just been through something crazy and have epinephrine rushing through your veins. So let your body sleep and regain its strength!

To wrap it up...

Having an allergic reaction can be a traumatizing experience that leaves you feeling uneasy, nervous, and not quite yourself. Realize that what you're feeling after a reaction is normal.

There are a few things you can do after a reaction to regroup. First, rest up. Sleep is good and, if you need to take some time off of school or work, that is totally understandable. When you're feeling a little better, it is a good idea to look back on the incident. Walk through exactly what happened and piece together what went wrong and how it was handled. Think about what you did and figure out if there is anything you would do differently. At the same time, it is also important to recognize what you did right. Maybe you took all the precautions you should have and the reaction happened due to something outside of your control. Maybe you did a really good job staying calm. Maybe you were good at communicating the fact that you were having a reaction. Maybe you gave yourself the auto-injector. Recognizing what you did well, and what you could do differently, will help you approach future situations.

Once you have taken time to think through the situation, and maybe talk it out with people you trust or an allergist, it is important not to dwell on it. Start moving forward with normal activities and your regular routine. And, with a bit of time, you will feel like yourself again.

Summary Tips

1) It's okay to feel "off" during the days immediately following a serious reaction.
2) Retrace your steps leading up to the reaction and think about how it could have been prevented.
3) Surround yourself with friends and family and share your feelings.

# Chapter 20
## *Being Confident with Food Allergies*

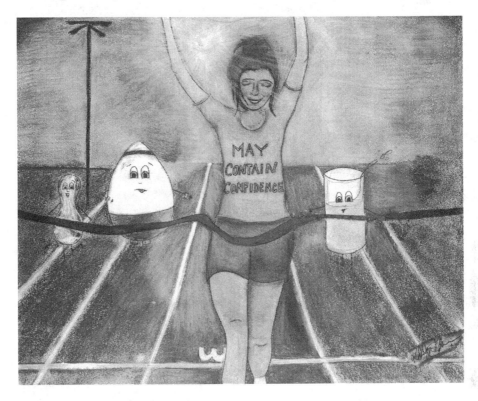

## Introduction

As a teen, it is common to try to fit in, prove yourself, be popular, and understand who you are. It's normal to struggle with confidence, too. Having food allergies can make it even more difficult because allergies can easily be perceived as a weakness or as something for which we should be sorry. Sometimes allergies can even feel like a burden to others.

Having confidence usually means accepting and liking yourself for who you are. But what's the secret to being okay with your allergies when they have mostly felt like a nuisance and an inconvenience for all of your life? Although sporting a "proud to be allergic" bumper sticker is a bit of a stretch, coming to terms with the reality that you have food allergies, and that they are an important part of you, yet don't define you, is a great attitude to have. This attitude can really help you balance safety with living a normal teenage life.

Aside from accepting your allergies as a part of you, being confident with your food allergies also comes with gains in knowledge and practice when it comes to dealing with different situations. Learning what you can about allergies, researching and planning ahead for new situations, and being open and straightforward about your allergies will be helpful when it comes to building your confidence.

## When things go right

### Learning the Hard Way, by Emily Rose

When I was in grade eight, I went to my first baseball game with my school. Before I went, my mom had talked to my teachers about my allergy. They decided it would be best to make me sit beside my teacher. My mom tried to prepare me with a lot of disinfectant before I went. I realized I was not prepared when we arrived. There were peanuts everywhere! My friends did not end up sitting beside me because I was with the teacher. I felt very alone and scared. To get through being scared, I just had to have confidence in myself and my abilities. I was very careful about what I touched and I did not eat anything. In the end, it all turned out okay. And now I know the severity of the situations I can handle alone.

### Accepting my Allergies, by Karen

I am a pretty outgoing person and I love to meet new people whenever I get the chance to. Entering university gave me the opportunity to meet so many new people and make new friends. Because I have a severe allergy, I knew this was also the opportunity to bring up my allergies early in friendships so there were no surprises later on. I was confident enough to introduce myself to new people and bring up my allergies as soon as I could (whether it was at a party or during a meal). The responses were reassuring.

For example, a friend of mine told me a story the other day about my food allergies. She was eating a peanut butter granola bar at her own house and there were crumbs on the floor. For some reason, she felt the need to pick up every little crumb off the floor in case I stepped on it and "decided to lick my foot" when I came over. This humorous example is a bit over the top, but the moral of the story here is that, even when I am not around, my friends are cautious about my allergies because I was confident enough to tell them about my allergies early on in our friendships.

**Treat your Allergies the way you want Others to Treat your Allergies, by Harrison**

I'm a 17 year old who is allergic to eggs, dairy, soy, seafood, nuts, apples, pears, and cherries. That's 8 things. And, when you count smaller foods that everyone ELSE can have such as candy (Halloween), cake (birthdays) or chocolates (Valentine's Day), it basically leaves me excluded from all of those special days. So that sucks. But, in a way, it doesn't. You see, I decided to treat my allergies the way I want others to treat my allergies. I flip allergies on their head in my own head and think that they are cool. I think auto-injectors are cool! What a cool, intricate device that is so simple. Yet it can also help save lives!

Taking some wisdom from one of my friends, and applying it to food allergies, you should have some fun with them. That's how I want others to see my allergies. I do not what people to see them as flaws I have or something to be embarrassed about. I often have fun with my allergies and say things like "I'm allergic to eggs, dairy, soy, seafood, nuts, apples, pears, cherries, and homework." I just try to sneak it in there for a bit of humour.

I figure that I'm likely to have my allergies for a long time. So I might as well accept them, have fun with them, and treat my allergies the way I want others to treat them—without any stigma attached to them and simply as a normal part of life.

## When things go wrong

### Cut Assumptions, not Corners, by Erika

I was attending a weekend leadership retreat away from home. We spent the weekend at a location where they ran camps during the summer and rented out cabins during the fall, winter, and spring months other groups. On our first day there, I spoke to the kitchen manager about my allergies, the severity of them, and the necessary precautions required to avoid cross-contamination. The kitchen manager assured me that everything would be okay. He went over the menu with me and cleared every meal.

On our first lunch, a server brought a salad dressing bottle, which he claimed was solely balsamic vinegar and olive oil, which I had asked for, since I was unable to have the regular dressing. I was deep in conversation with another leader and was confident that the head chef and kitchen staff had understood my allergies and that everything would go smoothly. I mean, it was just vinegar and oil. I poured it directly on the salad and had a very small bite. Immediately, I knew it was not vinegar and that they had given me soy sauce and olive oil instead of balsamic vinegar. I was lucky that, this time, the reaction was not severe. Once I had recovered, I went to the kitchen staff and explained what had happened. I asked to speak to the kitchen manager and head chef and asked them to pour a new bottle of vinegar and olive oil in front of me. I also asked if they could label it so I would get the same bottle for the next meals. They agreed and proceeded to fill a new bottle and write my name on it. I thanked them for doing so and returned to the cabin with my friends.

I reflected on what happened and knew that I had been too confident about the kitchen staff's ability to take my allergies seriously. I had trusted them more than I should have because everyone makes mistakes. I learned never to cut corners when it comes to my food allergies. I learned that I can never be too safe and that being too confident can be a risk.

*Quick Tip - Be wary when restaurant staff or chefs are overconfident when it comes to their abilities to handle your food allergies. Ask them a few questions just to make sure that their knowledge truly backs up their confidence.*

## What would you say? (Q&A)
*Dylan, Erika, and Giulia*

**Was there a particular age at which you became confident enough to speak for yourself at restaurants?**

**Dylan** - I think I was in grade 8 when I felt confident speaking for myself at restaurants. I knew that I would have more responsibility for my allergy when I entered high school and gained confidence before that to help prepare myself.

**Erika** - At age ten I became confident speaking for myself at restaurants. My parents had built up my confidence by having me ask the servers on my own. They were, of course, there to back me up if I forgot to mention an allergen or did not reinforce how serious my allergies were.

**Giulia** – Definitely as a teenager. Before high school, I would only go out with my parents. Entering high school, however, I had to learn how to speak up about my allergies on my own because I was going out with my friends more often.

**Why do you think it is tough to be confident with food allergies?**

**Dylan** - I find that, sometimes, food can be unpredictable. This can seem difficult and intimidating at first. But then I prepare myself, look into ingredients, and only eat something when I know for sure that the food is safe. If the food isn't safe, or if a voice inside me doesn't trust the food, I just avoid it and look elsewhere.

**Erika** - I believe it can sometimes be tough to be confident with food allergies because not everyone understands how serious and life-threatening food allergies can be. Often times their lack of awareness and knowledge can make me feel insecure about my own situation and others may make me feel like I am overreacting. This can make me lose confidence.

**Giulia** - I think it can sometimes be tough to be confident about your allergies because you are afraid of receiving bad news. For instance, it can be quite defeating to find out that you can't eat that cupcake that you wanted to try so badly.

**How do you overcome insecurities in different allergy-related situations?**

**Dylan** - I overcome insecurities by speaking up for myself. I find that a lot of my insecurities often lie within the ignorance others display about my food allergy. By speaking up and educating others, I can often create a better, allergy-safe environment around me.

**Erika** - When I feel insecure in allergy-related situations, I remind myself about the potential consequences if I do not speak up. I also think about times when being confident about who I am and trusting myself have helped me stay safe and avoid a reaction.

**Giulia** - I surround myself with people who understand my allergies. Their support helps me feel confident about myself and my insecurities tend not to emerge as often.

**Why is it so important to be confident with allergies and how can it be achieved?**

**Dylan** - I think my life would be more difficult if I weren't confident about allergies. With confidence in myself and about my allergies, I can do anything I've dreamed of doing without worrying that the world is out to get me! I achieve it through baby steps as I educate myself, my friends, and my family. Then I step out and challenge myself by educating teachers and restaurant staff. I don't think it's necessary to reach out to everyone. But I find that challenging myself in a safe environment, through learning, is rewarding and helps me gain confidence.

**Erika** - It is extremely important to be confident when living with food allergies because you are your own best advocate. And there will be times when you need to stand up for yourself. The keys to becoming more confident about your food allergies involve continuing to speak up about them, becoming knowledgeable about them, becoming knowledgeable about how reactions occur, and learning to trust yourself.

**Giulia** - If you're not confident, nobody around you will be confident about your ability to take care of yourself either. Confidence is key when it comes to getting people to respect you and understand you.

## To wrap it up...

Being confident about your food allergies involves two main challenges: One involves accepting your allergies as a part of who you are. The other involves learning how to manage your allergies in various situations.

It can be difficult to accept your allergies since they can seem like such a nuisance. However, if you read the next chapter, you'll see how teens with food allergies have learned to be thankful for what they have and even learned to appreciate some of the advantages (seriously!) of having food allergies.

Learning how to handle a variety of situations will also help you build confidence. In new situations, it is helpful to have others around you who know your allergies and how to handle a reaction.

When you surround yourself with people who "get it," you'll find it's easier to be confident in different situations. Furthermore, as you get more practice dealing with situations (such as dining out or travelling), you will become more and more confident.

## Summary Tips

1) Don't let allergies define you. There are many other things that make you, you.
2) Trust your gut and have faith in yourself and your years of experience with staying safe.
3) Practice the words you'll say in advance of certain tricky situations.

# Chapter 21

*Seeing the Bright Side*

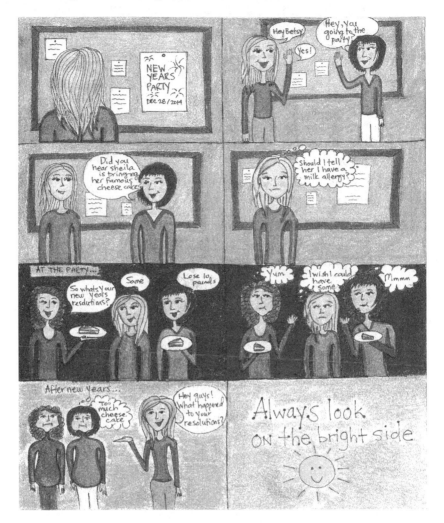

## Introduction

Having allergies can sometimes be a nuisance. Yet there are actually some surprising benefits. You've probably had people say things like "Wow, it must really suck not to be able to eat what everyone else is eating" or "Isn't it annoying having to carry around your auto-injector?" or "What CAN you even eat?" Sometimes it seems discouraging. But it is important to appreciate that being allergic is a part of who you are and that you can embrace it!

When talking to other teens with food allergies, the most common benefits of having allergies were thought to be greater maturity, a stronger sense of independence, and an appreciation for what we do have. Many teens have also made great friendships through meeting other people with allergies. And a lot of teens find that having allergies can give you fun conversation starters and crazy stories to share. It can also be very exciting when you find new foods you can eat or restaurants that are really good at handling your allergies. One teen said the following: "People that have allergies develop the ability to be observant, creative, and diligent while still living a normal life." Hopefully, by reading this chapter, you'll be able to think a bit about how allergies have actually had a positive impact on your life.

## When things go right

### Coming to Terms, by Chelsea

When I was young, I blamed my mom for giving me my allergy and ruining my life. This is harsh, I know. I felt like I could never reach my full potential and be who I wanted to be because my allergy was stopping me from doing it. Sometimes I felt like I didn't belong because of it. As I got older, I started to realize that it wasn't anyone's fault. Having an allergy was just a part of me and it wasn't necessarily a bad thing. I learned to accept people for their challenges and accept myself for mine. I found that, although an allergy wasn't something I would wish upon anyone, it is something that I have that I could use to help others—especially those with allergies. I've also found that it doesn't stop you from being who you want to be. Nor does it stop you from following your dreams as long as you want them badly enough.

### What's "Normal" Anyway, by Jazmin

Just like everyone else, I have my times when I think "Why do I have all these life-threatening allergies?" But I have learned that I have them for a reason. I am able to teach people about allergy safety and teach them new things that they might not have known about allergies. My allergies don't define me. But they are a part of my story and a part of who I am. I am grateful for what my allergies have taught me. I have learned things like compassion and caring towards others. But they have also taught me the realities and potential dangers in life. I have modified many recipes that often taste better (so I hear) than the originals. And I get to be a part of an amazing team of youth (I am a member of Food Allergy Canada's Youth Advisory Panel) that provides information to people all across the country. Some days are a struggle. But my allergies do not get me down. In fact, they do the opposite as they make me unique and different. Who wants to be normal anyway?

*Quick Tip* - *Try to think of three ways in which having allergies have actually made a positive impact upon your life. While having allergies is a nuisance, it's important to appreciate that there are actually some benefits.*

## When things go wrong

**Keeping Things in Perspective, by Talia**

I remember going to the children's hospital when I was younger to get allergy tests. Because I have so many different food allergies, I would get tested pretty often to see if I outgrew any or developed new ones. Although my mom tried to make the best out of the trips by buying me stuffed animals each time, I still hated it. I would get pricked and prodded, turn red and itchy, and then inevitably learn that I was still allergic to everything.

One day, after a particularly itchy appointment, I was in a sour mood. I was sulking and generally acting like a brat while my mom tried to soothe me. We were in the elevator on our way to leave the hospital when a little boy got on. His head was severely deformed and he looked pale and thin. I had to stop myself from staring. I realized that he was probably going through something much worse than I was. Although I didn't know what was wrong with him, I could tell it was serious.

Seeing that boy really put things in perspective for me. Having food allergies can be tough sometimes. But, by staying vigilant and safe, I can lead a normal and happy life. Allergies can suck sometimes. But they don't define who we are. It's important to concentrate on all the great things that we have in our lives as opposed to all of the negative things that can arise. Whenever I'm feeling down, I remind myself that there are people who have it much worse than I do and to be thankful for the amazing friends and family I've been blessed with to help me along the way.

**Staying Positive isn't Easy, by Erika**
I have been to many conferences, retreats, and camps. I always try to look on the bright side of my allergies. Having spent so much time away, I have learned to deal with my food allergies and have accepted that there will be meals or even activities that may make me feel left out or isolated. There are, however, always ways to change that. I have always tried to look on the bright side by telling myself that having food allergies has made me a more confident person. I have learned to speak up and be more responsible due to having to manage them and stay safe.

There have been times, however, when, even though I have tried to stay positive and focus on the "bright side of things," I have felt sad or frustrated about having to manage and cope with food allergies. Being able to see the positives in any given situation is important. Sometimes, though, that positive energy and thought is not nearly enough. We can feel down and a little left out. I have been to dinner parties where all I could eat were raw vegetables because we had not brought more food. The hosts had told me that everything would be safe for me. At these dinners, I told myself to focus on the facts that I could eat something, I was with friends and family, and that I could eat something when we returned home. Despite all of that positive thinking, I did feel upset. I felt upset that I had not brought a full "safe" meal for myself. I felt upset that the hosts did not understand my allergies. When "seeing the bright side of things" is not enough, I find it important to have friends and family there to support me and someone to talk to.

*Quick Tip - It's normal to feel down or frustrated about food allergies. Don't feel like you always must be overly positive in every situation and ignore your true emotions. Find out what is bothering you and try to deal with it for next time.*

## What would you say? (Q&A)
*Bailey, Lindsay and Stephanie*

**What is the best part about having allergies?**

**Bailey** - The best part about having allergies is getting to be part of a community where everyone is working to raise awareness about anaphylaxis. There's a sense of belonging and leadership within the Food Allergy Canada community which I am honoured to be a part of. Also, auto-injectors are pretty cool. Seriously. Not very many people just carry around a needle that can save their life!

**Lindsay** - Since my allergies usually lead me to not eating desserts, I always say that my allergies are keeping me healthy and saving me some unnecessary calories.

**Stephanie** - You are unique, you always have a conversation starter, and you are an "exception." Therefore, you are exceptional!

**Have you ever felt glad to have allergies?**

**Bailey** - There have been situations where I can honestly say that I was glad to have allergies. It's part of who I am and I've been able to meet some pretty awesome people because of it!

**Lindsay** - My allergies have inspired me to pursue a career in medicine. I hope to become an allergist. I am glad, therefore, that allergies are a part of my life. Otherwise I might not have arrived at that decision.

**Stephanie** - Once, one of my teachers brought small chocolates for our small group. Because she didn't know what was in the chocolates, she bought me a giant allergen-free chocolate bar. I was really glad to have allergies then (and my classmates wished they did too). I was also grateful for such a thoughtful teacher!

**If someone says "Wow, it must really suck to have allergies," what do you say back?**

**Stephanie** - It's not easy to have allergies. However, by informing others in advance and being careful, I can live a fulfilling and enjoyable life just like anyone else! I have plenty of variety and foods to choose from.

**Lindsay** - I respond by saying that it might suck sometimes. But it really doesn't limit me in anything that I do. I am still able to fully enjoy my life and live it how I want to even though I have allergies.

**Bailey** - The last time someone said "Wow it must really suck to have allergies" to me I was missing class to go to the allergist. So I responded with, "Wow it must really suck to have to go to math this afternoon."

**Would you be okay having allergies for the rest of your life?**

**Stephanie** - Yes, I have had allergies for over two decades and have learned to live with them. So I would be able to have them for the rest of my life. I may not have a choice. But, if you can't live without them, you may as well live well with them!

**Lindsay** - Having lived with my allergies my whole life, I would definitely be okay with having them for the rest of my years. I have accepted that it is highly unlikely that I will grow out of my allergies. So I am okay with having them forever.

**Bailey** - I would be okay with having food allergies for the rest of my life and, according to my allergist, I will likely have them for the rest of my life.

## To wrap it up...

Dealing with allergies is certainly challenging. And is not something we would wish upon anyone. However, taking a step back to appreciate the benefits to growing up with allergies can help you embrace them as part of who you are and help you to make the most of it.

Through reading this chapter, you've hopefully started to think about some of the positive impacts your allergies have had on you. Because of your allergies, maybe you were given a unique opportunity. Maybe you met some great friends. Maybe you can better appreciate how lucky you are in other ways. Maybe you have become more responsible and independent. Or maybe you have some great stories to tell. You have a unique challenge to face and you can use it to your advantage! So, the next time someone says to you, "Wow, it must really suck to have allergies," what are you going to say?

## Summary Tips

1) Remember that allergies are manageable and that they don't have to slow you down.
2) Never forget that you are an expert about a condition that even many adults don't know much about.
3) Keep things in perspective and be thankful for all of the good things in your life.

## Conclusion

This book has covered so much on situations, emotions and what living with allergies is truly like. The stories and advice throughout share positives and negatives for living with food allergies. It's not always an easy road, but always remember that it's a road that many have travelled successfully down before. Stay confident, surround yourself with people who respect you and your allergies, and never take chances with your allergies.

You know how to stay safe with your allergies. But with so many other influences like peer pressure, anxiety, friends, assumptions, appearances and more affecting decisions, slip-ups can happen. Trust your gut and know that you truly are an expert on living with a condition that even many adults don't know much about. Have faith in yourself and your abilities. Stay positive and define your allergies, don't let them define you.

If you are ever looking to connect with other teens with allergies, or looking for more information, contact Food Allergy Canada (formerly Anaphylaxis Canada). We're always here to help.